HUMAN SUBJECTS IN MEDICAL EXPERIMENTATION

HEALTH, MEDICINE, AND SOCIETY:
A WILEY-INTERSCIENCE SERIES

DAVID MECHANIC, Editor

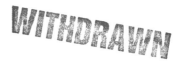

BRADFORD H. GRAY

HUMAN SUBJECTS IN MEDICAL EXPERIMENTATION

A Sociological Study of the Conduct
and Regulation of Clinical Research

A WILEY-INTERSCIENCE PUBLICATION

JOHN WILEY & SONS, New York • London • Sydney • Toronto

Library of Congress Cataloging in Publication Data

Gray, Bradford H   1942–
    Human subjects in medical experimentation.

    (Health, medicine, and society)
    "A Wiley-Interscience publication."
    Includes bibliographical references and index.
    1. Human experimentation in medicine.   I. Title.
[DNLM: 1. Ethics, Medical.   2. Human experimentation.
3. Research. W20.5 G778h]

R853.H8G7   174'.2   74-20638

Printed in the United States of America

10 9 8 7 6 5 4 3 2 1

FOR ANNE

FOREWORD

I take great pleasure in introducing an important new talent in medical sociology. As the reader will soon see, Bradford Gray's book not only speaks to an important matter of current social policy; it is also a model study soundly based on sociological theory and research methods. Indeed, its systematic data on human subjects' knowledge and feelings about being subjects, and on the actual process of peer review committee decisions about research protocols using human subjects, are unique in the rapidly growing literature on the ethics of the use of human subjects in biomedical research.

There is no need, with a book so well organized, so lucidly stated, so well argued, to rehearse its author's findings, conclusions, and recommendations for policy change. The book has an almost dramatic structure that will carry the reader along from his research procedures through to his conclusions and recommendations. I merely want to bring out and thereby stress one implicit point that Dr. Gray, thoroughgoing sociologist that he is, has perhaps left a bit more understated than it should be.

The fact is that Gray is not describing a particular case in which a few delinquent researchers have failed to live up to satisfactory ethical standards for the medical profession. He is analyzing a system of social relationships which, because of its improvable defects as a system, can and should be changed so that the individuals who participate in that system can better fulfill the high ethical standards that medical researchers profess. There is a mistaken belief held by some medical researchers, and even by those who deplore the defects in present practices in this field, that the shortcomings and scandals that occur can be traced to a handful of individuals who lack the requisite personal qualities. They recommend that "the honest, conscientious, compassionate physician" be the "ultimate" safeguard of the human research subject. But Gray's book shows that "honest, conscientious, compassionate" physicians have been led into bad practice by a bad system. He reveals to us a review committee that was not active enough, principal investigators too busy being scientists to give adequate value and attention to the ethical aspects of their research, and the lack of adequate informal peer control in the daily research situation. It is the system of social relationships that needs changing, he shows, though of course he assumes that such a changed system depends on the recruitment of, and will itself continuously help to create, "honest, conscientious, compassionate physicians."

During the last 35 years or so, the great excitement and rewards in medical research have been on the scientific side, rather than on the ethical side that our marvelous scientific progress has brought into ever greater importance. Does not the medical research profession now need to transfer some of the initiative, energy, and concern that it shows in science to the ethical problems that science creates? Not the least virtue of Gray's book is that it provides needed knowledge and guidance for this neglected task.

BERNARD BARBER
Professor of Sociology
Barnard College and Columbia University

The completion of a long-term project leaves one acutely aware of the many contributions of others who made it possible. My greatest debt is to two medical researchers (who I agreed not to identify by name) who allowed me to interview their research subjects. Even though my questions potentially reflected upon the performance of an important aspect of their dealings with research subjects—the matter of informed consent—these investigators not only gave me their permission to talk to their subjects, but actively cooperated with me and assisted me in every way I requested. In addition, the principal investigator in the labor-induction study offered a number of useful suggestions in response to an earlier draft of this book. I am also indebted to the research staff in the two projects, whose day-to-day assistance was essential to the completion of my interviews.

Gathering the data for this study also required the cooperation of the research subjects in the two projects studied and interviews with 13 medical researchers whose projects did not become the focus of this study. All of these people gave me at least an hour of their time, for which I could offer only my gratitude.

The final anonymous source to be acknowledged is the chairman of the Clinical Research Committee. His interest in my project and active cooperation in making available to me the records of the committee were of key importance to this study.

This book is a revision of my doctoral dissertation at Yale University for which my principal advisors were August B. Hollingshead, Jerome K. Myers, and Raymond S. Duff. The research was supported in part by National Institute of Mental Health training grant MH-10340. My original interest in this area was stimulated by Diana Crane in her seminar in sociology of science at Yale. I am also grateful to Jay Katz of the Yale Law School and Robert J. Levine of the Yale School of Medicine for their encouragement and advice at several stages of this project. The interest of my friend Stephen Kunitz, now of University of Rochester School of Medicine, was of great value, as were his comments and suggestions on one draft of this book.

While planning this study, I spent some time with the Research Group on Human Experimentation at Columbia University—Bernard Barber, John Lally, Julia Makarushka, and Daniel Sullivan. They were gathering the data for their book, *Research on Human Subjects* (Russell Sage, 1973), and gave me the benefit of their experience to that point. Although our projects were not coordinated with each other, I believe that they dovetail in many ways. I owe a special debt to Bernard Barber who responded enthusiastically to my dissertation and urged me to revise it for publication. He has been an invaluable source of advice as I worked on the manuscript to prepare it for publication.

I would also like to thank David Mechanic, the academic editor of Health, Medicine, and Society: A Wiley-Interscience Series, for his highly useful and detailed comments on the next to last draft of this book. I am also indebted to Eric Valentine, my editor at Wiley-Interscience, for shepherding the book into print, and to Christine Valentine, who edited the manuscript. Sherry Brandt provided superior proofreading assistance.

Mrs. Lillian Smith typed the questionnaires used in the data gathering; Janet Turk lent her expert editorial pencil to the first version of the first two chapters; Janet Jensen, Susan Morton, Rosalie Radcliffe, Robin Ratliff, Sally Rogers, Addie Spangler, and Shelby Tucker typed all or part of various drafts; and the staff of the Institute for Research in Social Science at the University of North Carolina assisted with the data analysis. My colleague, John Shelton Reed, made several useful suggestions regarding the presentation of some of the results.

Finally, I would like to acknowledge those to whom my debts are not specific to this book.

To Richard F. Larson, then of Oklahoma State University and now of California State University at Hayward, I would again like to express my gratitude for support and encouragement at a crucial time in my early professional development.

To my parents, who have long shown interest and pride in my work.

To my wife, Anne, and my children, Carrie and Joshua, for making my life so happy.

With such extensive debts for the assistance of so many people, it is apparent that the ultimate responsibility for errors and shortcomings is my own.

BRADFORD H. GRAY

University of North Carolina, Chapel Hill
July 1974

ACKNOWLEDGMENTS

For permission to reproduce quotations from published works, grateful acknowledgment is made to the following: to Anna Freud for "The Doctor-Patient Relationship"; to Henry K. Beecher and Little, Brown & Company for *Research and the Individual* (copyright 1970 by Little, Brown); to *Annals of Internal Medicine* for "The Doctor Himself as a Therapeutic Agent" by W. R. Houston; to the *New England Journal of Medicine* for "Physician and Patient as a Social System" by L. J. Henderson (Vol. 212, pp. 819–823, 1935); to Maurice B. Visscher and the *Annals of the New York Academy of Science* for "The Two Sides of the Coin in the Regulation of Experimental Medicine"; to *Daedalus,* Journal of the American Academy of Arts and Sciences, Boston, Massachusetts, for exerpts from articles by Stephen Graubard, Hans Jonas, Hermann Blumbart, Paul Freund, Guido Calabresi, Louis Jaffe, and Jay Katz in the Spring 1969 issue, *Ethical Aspects of Experimentation with Human Subjects,* and for quotations by Geoffrey Edsall and Walsh McDermott from the November 1967 Conference on the Ethical Aspects of Experimentation on Human Subjects; to Aldine Publishing Company for *Prescription for Leadership* by Stephen J. Miller; to Michael E. De Bakey and the *Journal of the American Medical Association* for "Medical Research and the Golden Rule"; to the William B. Eerdmans Publishing Company for "The Law of Genetic Therapy" by Alexander Capron in *The New Genetics and the Future of Man*; to the Russell Sage Foundation for *Experimentation with Human Beings,* edited by Jay Katz (copyright 1972 by Russell Sage Foundation).

B. H. G.

CONTENTS

TABLES

CHAPTER ONE

THE ETHICS AND REGULATION
OF HUMAN EXPERIMENTATION

Although the use of human beings as experimental subjects in biomedical and behavioral research has emerged as a topic of great interest and concern in the past decade, surprisingly little empirical research has been done on the conduct of this fascinating and complex activity. This book is a sociologist's study of some aspects of human experimentation in medicine. It is based in great part on interviews with the subjects of two research projects conducted in a major university's medical center, and thus offers a new window through which to view experimentation on human beings.

The issues raised by human experimentation have become more widely recognized, though perhaps not better understood, through the prominent news coverage given to such recent dramatic cases as the deliberate infection with hepatitis of institutionalized mentally retarded children at Willowbrook in New York State, Defense Department sponsored whole-body radiation of cancer patients at the University of Cincinnati Medical School, brain surgery to modify the behavior of incarcerated individuals in Michigan and California, and the Tuskegee study of syphilis among men from whom treatment was withheld.[1] It should not be assumed that most ethically problematic research makes the news, however; both reason and considerable evidence suggest that most instances go unreported. Nevertheless, the cases that have been brought to light have heightened public concern, and several Congressional committees have become interested in matters of ethics and research. In September 1973 the U.S. Senate voted 81 to 6 in favor of a bill establishing a National Commission for the Protection of Human Subjects of Biomedical and Behavioral Research.[2] This commission is to develop guidelines for the conduct of such research and policies for assuring that subjects' rights are fully protected.*

Even without such a commission, however, the problems involved in human experimentation will almost certainly receive active attention in future years. They are part of the very nature of research activities which have great recognized value and societal support. Ethical problems cannot be evaded even by abolishing human experimentation—which no one seriously proposes—because the failure to pursue knowledge that might benefit mankind may itself be unethical. Furthermore, the distinction between experimentation and therapy can be most problematic. It is often asserted that because individual variations among patients are so great, any "therapeutic" intervention (or nonintervention) is "experimental" because the outcome in any given patient cannot be predicted with certainty. In a more concrete example, expert witnesses before the Senate Subcommittee on Health recently disagreed about whether psychosurgery, that is, brain surgery for the purpose of modifying behavior, is experimental. This difficulty in reliably distinguishing between experimental and nonexperimental procedures is one factor that has led some thoughtful commentators to suggest that the rules which apply in the "experimental" situation—for example, that risk should be outweighed by potential benefits, and the requirement for "informed consent"—should apply to all situations, whether "experimental" or "therapeutic." Whatever the merits of this argument, the issues presented by human experimentation are clearly not issues we can avoid.

In addition, the ethical issues in human experimentation defy definitive solution. That is, even though certain general principles and guidelines can be widely agreed upon as sound, their application to actual cases will necessarily be interpretive and subjective. For example, a basic ethical principle in biomedical research is that the risks to the subjects of an experiment must be outweighed by its potential benefits, either to the subjects, to future patients, or to "science." However, people who are in complete agreement about the validity of this principle may nevertheless be unable to agree about whether the risk/benefit ratio in a given piece of research is sufficiently low to justify its conduct. Risks and benefits cannot be measured with a device independent of the measurer. What we do is to establish a procedure and declare it to be the solution to the problem. Thus, committees have been created to make the judgments that are inherent in the application of general principles to concrete cases. While this procedure avoids some of the conflict-of-interest problems that arise when an investi-

* A revised version of this bill subsequently passed both houses and was signed into law in July 1974.

gator proceeds solely on the basis of his own assessment of the risk/benefit ethicality of his research, it is still likely that a committee's decisions will to some extent reflect its composition, the procedures that it follows, its work load at a particular time, and other factors that are irrelevant to the issue of whether the risks are, in fact, outweighed by the benefits. The basic question remains unsolved. No definitive answer is possible to the question of how high a probability of achieving how much benefit from a piece of research is necessary to justify exposing X number of human subjects to Y levels of risk.

Critics of current practices in the conduct of human experimentation commonly begin or end by discussing the beneficial knowledge that has resulted from research.[3] At first this seems odd, since the audience for such writings can scarcely be unaware of such benefits. Nor can such statements be dismissed as a dodge used by individuals who are really opposed to human experimentation but who know that an argument made by someone who is obviously hostile to research would get scant attention from researchers and policy makers. The fact is that some of the most serious criticisms have come from individuals who have solid credentials as researchers. The aim has clearly not been to stop research, although strong arguments have been made that certain types of research (such as psychosurgery for some purposes and research involving live, aborted fetuses) should be temporarily or permanently halted or that certain categories of subjects (such as prisoners or mentally retarded) should not be used for some or all kinds of research. Rather, the thrust of the criticisms is that human experimentation is an important activity of great societal benefit that must be conducted in a manner consistent with basic societal beliefs and values about the rights and worth of the individual. While this society has been willing to support substantial research activities, the result of public attention to research that grossly violates our ethical sensibilities has often been the imposition of additional controls over the conduct of such research.

Perhaps it is the conflict between two strongly felt values—support for research and the upholding of our concepts of individual rights and dignity—that makes the topic so fascinating. The dramatic risks and benefits of some research must add to the attraction as well. Contributions to the discussion of the issues have come from such disparate fields as theology,[4] philosophy,[5] the law,[6] the social sciences,[7] journalism,[8] and medicine,[9] and the conflict between values is a recurrent theme. A number of conceptualizations for this conflict have been offered: individual rights versus societal rights,[10] the right balance between present lives and future lives,[11] individual morality and statistical morality,[12] immediate benefits versus future benefits,[13] the dilemma of science and therapy.[14] Perhaps the most intriguing formulation comes from Guido Calabresi:

> there is a deep conflict between our fundamental need constantly to reaffirm our belief in the sanctity of life and our practical placing of some values (including future lives) above an individual life. That conflict suggests, at the very least, the need for a quite complex structuring to enable us *sometimes* to sacrifice lives, but hardly ever to do it blatantly and as a society, and above all to allow this sacrifice under quite rigid controls.[15]

In the face of this conflict, however conceptualized, the usual goal is to resolve the ethical and legal issues without inhibiting the quest for new knowledge, to protect the individual subject's rights and welfare while encouraging research activities that may have widespread societal benefit.

Little recognition has been given to the possibility that the two values cannot be simultaneously maximized. A statement by a researcher with whom I am acquainted illustrates the point. He wanted me to look at a consent form he had prepared for subjects in a study he was undertaking. His hope, he said, was that the form would contain all of the ethically required information concerning risks, alternatives, and so forth, but that the full communication of this material would not result in any potential subjects refusing to participate in the study. The governmental policies that have been developed in this area reflect the same understandable desire. However, whether it is possible to devote more extensive efforts to guaranteeing the ethicality and legality of human experimentation without making it more difficult to recruit subjects and to follow rigorous experimental designs is an important question that will have to be faced. Should it become apparent that the maintaining of certain ethical standards effectively slows research, the depth of societal commitment to the relevant values of individual worth will be put to a stronger test than has yet been faced.

THE PRESENT STUDY

The question of whether a more rigorous application of ethical standards will inhibit research is only one of the many empirical questions about human experimentation about which little or no data exist. Most of the literature in this area stems from reflections based on personal experiences or from expertise in philosophy, theology, or the law. My belief that more systematically gathered information on the actual conduct of human experimentation would be useful to the continuing discussions of the issues was one factor that prompted this study. Important policies regulating human experimentation have been implemented, even though systematic information about existing practices was sparce. In particular, very little is known about such vital matters as how subjects are selected, their characteristics, the process through which they come to be involved, and the reasons why they participate.

All of this is to say that the perspective of the research subject has been largely missing from the dialogue on human experimentation. Thus, I devoted much of my effort to what could be learned with subjects in two projects at a large university's medical center. Additional data came from records, interviews with researchers, and observations of the daily conduct of medical research in that setting.

In part, then, this book is about the ways people become involved in research and the reasons why they become subjects. Depending upon the nature of the study, the risks taken by subjects may be negligible, high, or even unknown, and the research may or may not have the intent of directly benefiting them. Subjects' reasons for volunteering for research that has immediate therapeutic intent seem to be apparent, particularly in situations in which nonexperimental alternatives do not exist or are unpromising. This book, however, is about two studies in which such obvious motivational factors *cannot* explain subjects' participation. What did explain their participation in a substantial number of cases was ignorance of the research or feelings of constraint which prevented their refusal. These aspects of the research situation will be examined in detail.

This book can also be seen as a partial assessment of current governmental policies regulating the use of human subjects in medical research.[16] The experiences of Nazi Germany made it apparent that the "experimental" use of human beings could be monstrously perverted,[17] and raised the worldwide concern that led to efforts both to fix responsibility and to design rules that would prevent the recurrence of such horrors. The 1960s in the United States found such concerns about human experimentation arising in a context of increasing governmental support for medical research. The result was a decision by the U.S. Public Health Service (PHS) to require medical research institutions to establish peer review committees to oversee the conduct of human experimentation. It was hoped that these committees would prevent the unethical and even illegal use of human subjects such as had come to light in the United States in the previous several years. This book is a case study of the functioning of that peer review procedure and an examination of its adequacy—and its inadequacy—for protecting the health and rights of human subjects. Data from one such peer review committee as well as data from research subjects will be used in this regard.

Along these same lines, I also hope that this book will provide useful case study material of problems of social control in professions. Social control is an interesting problem in professions, because these occupations are characterized by a particularly high degree of autonomy. As Freidson[18] has pointed out, this freedom from outside control is based on the claim that professional work is of such a high intellectual or technical nature as to render laymen largely incapable of regulating or evaluating it intelligently. It is based upon the further assertions that professionals are trained to be responsible and do not require supervision to perform at a highly competent or ethical level, and that proper regulatory action can be entrusted to the profession itself should individual practitioners prove not to be responsible. The PHS's required *peer* review procedure is consistent with these notions since such committees are controlled by medical researchers, although the regulations most recently proposed by the Department of Health, Education, and Welfare state that they should include persons who are capable of assessing proposed research from the standpoint of "applicable law" and "community attitudes."[19]

The social control problems in human experimentation result from the fact that the securing of ethically necessary informed consent of subjects often requires no little effort by researchers. Furthermore, complete disclosure may appear to be against an investigator's immediate interests, because it may be feared that the probability of a subject's agreeing to participate may be reduced if he understands the risks of and alternatives to being an experimental subject. Evidence from this study suggests that the present primary reliance on the before-the-fact social control devices of professional socialization and peer review of proposed research is not sufficient to insure that investigators will conduct research only if they have the informed consent of their subjects. In the professions as elsewhere, the lack of visibility of an individual's behavior and the absence of devices to detect "deviant behavior" can lead to a casual attitude toward strictly proper behavior. If detection is not likely, all one need satisfy is one's conscience. While conscience is no doubt an effective restraint in many instances, it can be avoided all too easily by one form or another of self-deception. In medical research this can result in the participation of subjects who have not, in any meaningful sense, given their informed consent.

Finally, this study provides some description of the daily realities of two rather ordinary medical research projects conducted in a large university medical center. Medical research is often thought of in terms of the dramatic, life-saving advances that capture the attention of the mass media and the public. However, medical research is more typically a rather routine and unglamorous enterprise, comprised mainly of small studies that make minute contributions to medical knowledge and are published in a staggering number of professional journals. A great deal of print has been devoted to the sensational (such as heart transplants) and the scandalous (such as the Tuskegee syphilis studies), but little is known of the daily reality of medical research. The present study suggests that medical research, like so much other work, can be routine and repetitive.

As findings are presented, I also suggest that some commonly held notions about human experimentation—and policies based on those notions—are of questionable general validity and are completely misleading in some situations. I raise questions about such matters as the concept of the "volunteer" as a maker of decisions regarding himself, about the notion that a concerned, conscientious physician-researcher is the best protector of the research subject,[20] about the concept of informed consent and the use of written "consent forms," and about the nature of the researcher-subject relationship.

The remainder of this chapter is devoted to two other matters that provide context for the results of this investigation: a brief review of current standards of ethics regarding the use of human subjects, and a description of the procedures required by the Public Health Service for protecting subjects' rights and welfare.

ETHICS OF HUMAN EXPERIMENTATION

The ethics of human experimentation have been formalized into at least thirty-three different guidelines and codes of ethics since World War II.[21] However, five relatively simple basic principles appear to be generally accepted. A research subject must be a person who volunteered on the basis of having all the necessary information for his decision to be an informed one. He should be allowed to withdraw from the research at whatever point he wishes. All unnecessary risks should be eliminated in the design of the research and through prior animal experimentation. The benefits of the experiment, either to the subject or to society should outweigh the risks to the subject. Finally, an experiment should be conducted only by individuals qualified to do so. These basic elements are embodied in such important codes as the Nuremberg Code (1946–1949), the Declaration of Helsinki (revised 1964), the AMA Code (1966), and U.S. Public Health Service requirements (December 12, 1966).[22]

There has been relatively little disagreement about the validity of these general principles. They do, however, contain and conceal several problems. For example, as mentioned before, their application in actual practice is bedeviled by various ambiguities and opportunities for interpretation. In addition, there are situations that contain ethical dilemmas that go beyond the simple principles just mentioned, the most frequent ones probably being research involving persons such as children who may be unable to give informed consent, and research that uses captive populations such as prisoners, for whom freedom to refuse to participate is a matter of concern.

The question of whether an experimental intervention is intended to benefit (therapeutically or diagnostically) its subjects is an additional complicating factor. Not only is the question itself difficult to resolve in some cases, but it has important implications for the issues of risk/benefit and informed consent. A study that is intended to have direct benefit for its subjects has fewer problems from the standpoint of risk/benefit, but it also involves some special ambiguities regarding requirements for disclosure, particularly of risks. It has been observed that there is a "traditional but largely unexamined prerogative of professionals to intervene in their patients' behalf without full disclosure whenever it is supposed to be 'in their patients' best interests.'"[23] Thus, patient benefit can cloud the disclosure requirements in an experiment, as can be seen in the current Department of Health, Education, and Welfare (DHEW) policy on protection of human subjects:

> Where an activity involves therapy, diagnosis, or management, and a professional/patient relationship exists, it is necessary "to recognize that each patient's mental and emotional condition is important . . . and that in discussing the element of risk, a certain amount of discretion must be employed consistent with full disclosure of fact necessary to any informed consent."[24]

Research that involves no benefit to its subjects may raise particularly vexing questions regarding risk/benefit (for example, Can exposure to significant risk ever be outweighed solely by additions to scientific knowledge?), but there are no ambiguities regarding disclosure. Full disclosure is required, as the same DHEW document makes clear:

> Where an activity does not involve therapy, diagnosis, or management, and a professional/subject rather than a professional/patient relationship exists, "the subject is entitled to a full and frank disclosure of all the facts, probabilities, and opinions which a reasonable man might be expected to consider before giving his consent."[25]

An important characteristic of the two research projects studied here is that peer review of both projects effectively resolved these issues and left the practical ethical requirements relatively clear and simple. The need for informed consent, with full disclosure, was unambiguous, and all subjects were adult, conscious, and free (that is, not prisoners). Thus, we will be talking about two studies in which there was the clear requirement of full disclosure by investigators and informed consent from the subjects themselves (not their representatives). It will be shown that even though both studies were conducted in accordance with existing Public Health Service procedures regarding the use of human subjects, serious shortcomings did exist in the extent to which informed consent was actually obtained. The factors responsible for this are examined in considerable detail in this book, because they are general problems that exist in much clinical research being done today.

THE REGULATION OF HUMAN EXPERIMENTATION

Formal procedures for the protection of the rights and welfare of most human subjects are a recent development, although recognition of the complex legal and ethical issues raised by the necessity to use human beings as research subjects is hardly new. Legal concern with human experimentation goes as far back as 1767 when an English court wrote that "many men very skillful in their profession have frequently acted out of the common way for the sake of trying experiments . . . they have acted ignorantly and unskillfully, contrary to the known rule and usage of surgeons."[26] The dangers of doing harm to human subjects were written of by the great nineteenth century French experimentalist, Claude Bernard.[27] In 1833 the famous American investigator William Beaumont, in his writings on the need for human experimentation when information is not otherwise available, mentioned the importance of methodological soundness so that subjects are not exposed to risks for no scientific benefit. He also pointed out the need for voluntary consent and the necessity to discontinue a project "when the subject becomes dissatisfied."[28]

The actual conduct of human experimentation has been an object of criticism for at least half a century. In memoirs translated from Russian and published in 1916,[29] the physician Veressayev wrote heatedly about "experiments on man." He focused particularly on a series of experiments in which the nature and mode of transmission of gonorrhea and syphilis were investigated by inoculating human subjects with discharges taken from patients with those diseases. He cited experiments published in many countries, including Britain and the United States, and concluded that "it is high time . . . for society to take its own measures of self-protection against those zealots of science who have ceased to distinguish between their brothers and guinea pigs, without waiting for the faculty to emerge from its lethargy."[30] The research he described differs little in purpose from the recently revealed experiments in which a group of Southern black men with syphilis were left untreated for more than 25 years after successful therapy for the disease was discovered, in order that long-term effects of the disease could better be studied.[31]

But it was Nazi Germany that brought all the difficult issues involved in human experimentation to the fore. As Stephen Graubard put it:

> It would be difficult to overstate the impetus this uniquely tragic European experience gave to studies of the ethics of human experimentation. Out of concern with the violence done to human beings came an interest in defining precisely the conditions under which human experimentation might take place.[32]

These concerns were felt by American medicine at the same time as biomedical research was expanding through an unprecedented level of support from the federal government and other sources. The National Institutes of Health (NIH) budget, for example, rose from less than half a million dollars prior to World War II, to around two and a half million by 1945, to 29 million in 1948, to more than 738 million in 1962, to almost one and a quarter billion in 1966.[33] Thus, the issues were raised in most dramatic and tragic form at the beginning of the period in which they would become more important statistically than ever before. By 1970, NIH awarded grants for more than 3000 projects that involved human subjects.[34]

An important step in federal involvement in the conduct of human experimentation came in the 1962 Drug Amendments Act,[35] which followed in the wake of the Thalidomide tragedy. This bill, also known as the Kefauver-Harris bill, made several important changes in the regulation of the ethical drug industry. Most important in the present context was the requirement that the Food and Drug Administration (FDA) impose new regulations on the clinical testing of experimental drugs. These regulations were to include the mandatory requirement of informed consent, with two poorly defined exceptions—investigators using investigational drugs were required to certify to the sponsor or manufacturer that they would "inform any human beings to whom such drugs, or any controls used in connection therewith, are being administered, or their representatives, that such drugs are being used for investigational purposes and will obtain the consent of such human beings or their representatives, except where they deem it not feasible or, in their professional judgment, contrary to the best interests of such human beings."[36] Over the years these exceptions became more carefully defined and limited. It is highly likely, however, that rationalizations such as not wanting to "upset" a patient's "well-being" were used in many cases to justify an investigator's failure to seek genuine informed consent from subjects.[37]

As Curran has pointed out,[38] these FDA regulations had two major limitations: they did not cover all aspects of subject protection since they were limited to the administration of investigational drugs, and the substantive requirement of informed consent was instituted without the establishment of any procedural requirements. The most important procedural requirements were to come later, in 1966, from the agency that was responsible for providing the funds for a large share of the nation's medical research—the National Institutes of Health and its parent, U.S. Public Health Service. It was these requirements that provided the regulatory framework under which the medical research projects I studied were conducted.

PUBLIC HEALTH SERVICE POLICY

Regulations set forth by the U.S. Public Health Service (and more recently by the Department of Health, Education, and Welfare) constitute the primary procedural requirements now existing for the protection of the rights and welfare of human research subjects in the United States.[39] Early PHS involvement in regulating the use of human subjects was associated with the opening of the National Institutes of Health Clinical Center in 1953. The need was recognized for principles and procedures to protect subjects, and a policy document, called "Group Consideration of Clinical Research Procedures Deviating From Accepted Medical Practice or Involving Unusual Hazard," was issued in November, 1953.[40] This document showed particular concern with the issue of acceptable risks to subjects and with what should be disclosed to subjects; it also introduced the idea that such issues in any particular project should be subjected to group consideration. However, primary responsibility for the conduct of clinical investigation remained with principal investigators. These original guidelines were revised in 1966, but continued to pertain only to "intramural programs" of the PHS.

In February 1966, the Surgeon General announced the beginning of PHS requirements to regulate the use of human subjects in "extramural research," that is, research supported by grants, contracts, and awards from the PHS and done in such settings as medical schools and teaching hospitals. Over the years it had become apparent that the lack of written guidelines had led to the absence of any uniformity of practice regarding human subjects in PHS-supported research. For example, Mark Frankel reports the recollection of Dr. James Shannon, director of NIH from 1955–1968, of an early, unsuccessful effort to transplant an animal kidney into a human being. This experiment was performed at a university hospital by a surgeon who consulted with no one about the procedure which, in

Shannon's words, "had neither likelihood of therapeutic benefit to the patient nor likelihood of providing new scientific information."[41]

The existence of the general problem of lack of uniformity and control over human experimentation was also evident in the results of a 1962 study[42] commissioned by NIH. This survey of university departments of medicine found no trend toward the establishment of policies for clinical research. The atmosphere of concern which led to the creation of the PHS regulations was also affected in the early 1960s by the increased general awareness of the issues in clinical research, which resulted from the development of statements on human experimentation by the World Medical Association (the "Declaration of Helsinki") and the Medical Research Council of Great Britain.

Thus, for several years prior to the development of PHS regulations to protect human subjects there had been in PHS some concern and awareness of general problems in the use of human subjects. Although this atmosphere was important, it was probably the occurrence of a major scandal in human experimentation that resulted in concrete steps being taken by PHS early in 1966. Eminent researchers with the Sloan-Kettering Cancer Foundation injected live cancer cells under the skin of uninformed subjects. The case, when it came to light, created great public furor, and eventually resulted in the researchers being found guilty of charges of unethical conduct and being censured and placed on probation.[43] The notoriety of this case provided the final impetus leading to the creation of the PHS policy to regulate the use of human subjects in research.[44]

Receiving less public attention, but of great importance within the medical research community, were the revelations made by Harvard professor Henry Beecher in a 1966 article in the *New England Journal of Medicine,* in which he reviewed published accounts of 22 "unethical or questionably ethical studies."[45] Although the PHS guidelines were already in final stages of preparation when the Beecher article was published, this article may well have smoothed the way for acceptance of the guidelines since it made a convincing case of the need for some kind of regulation. Beecher's credentials as a researcher and the prestige of the journal that printed his thoroughly documented article must have added to the legitimacy and impact of his charges within the research community.

The requirements instituted by the PHS in 1966[46] were based on the following general policy:

> Public Health Service support of clinical research and investigation involving human beings should be provided only if the judgment of the investigator is subject to prior review by his institutional associates to assure an independent determination of the protection of the rights and welfare of the individual or indi-

viduals involved, of the appropriateness of the methods used to secure informed consent, and of the risks and potential medical benefits of the investigation.[47]

The resulting PHS requirements—which were essentially unchanged when the field work for this study was done in the fall of 1970 and spring of 1971—can be briefly summarized as follows. The PHS required institutions in which PHS funds provided support for research involving human subjects (virtually all institutions doing medical research in the United States) to establish committees to review proposed research prior to submission to PHS for funding. Such committees were to assure that the "rights and welfare" of subjects would be protected, to judge the appropriateness of proposed procedures for securing informed consent, and to assess the risks and benefits of the research. The composition of the committee was not closely specified other than it was to include "staff of, or consultants to, [the] institution who are at the same time acquainted with the investigator under review, free to assess his judgment without placing in jeopardy their own goals, and sufficiently mature and competent to make the necessary assessment."[48] Originally it was left up to each institutional committee to "determine what constitutes the rights and welfare of human subjects in research, what constitutes informed consent, and what constitutes the risks and benefits of a particular investigation."[49] Later statements and clarifications provided more guidance in these areas. These review committees were also charged with providing a continuing review of projects, but this meant little more than asking investigators to apprise their peer review committee when modifications were made in previously approved projects. Finally, the institutional peer review committees were required to keep documentation of their reviews and records of informed consent.

Such were the general peer review requirements, as stated in PHS policy documents, at the time this study was begun in 1970. In Chapter Three I will describe how these general requirements were translated into practice by one large and very busy peer review committee.

It may be useful to note one further development in governmental policy in this area since the field work for the present study was done, and to point out some important limitations to this policy. In 1971, the *Institutional Guide to DHEW Policy on Protection of Human Subjects* was published. It contained considerably more detail than had earlier PHS policy statements.[50] For example, informed consent was defined more carefully:

Informed consent is the agreement obtained from a subject, or from his authorized representative, to the subject's participation in an activity.

The basic elements of informed consent are:

1. A fair explanation of the procedures to be followed, including an identification of those which are experimental;
2. A description of the attendant discomforts and risks;
3. A description of the benefits to be expected;
4. A disclosure of appropriate alternative procedures that would be advantageous for the subject;
5. An offer to answer any inquiries concerning the procedures;
6. An instruction that the subject is free to withdraw his consent and to discontinue participation in the project or activity at any time.

In addition, the agreement, written or oral, entered into by the subject, should include no exculpatory language through which the subject is made to waive, or to appear to waive, any of his legal rights, or to release the institution or its agents from liability for negligence.[51]

The DHEW *Institutional Guide* also required that the review of proposed projects by institutional committees should "determine the acceptability of the proposal in terms of institutional commitments and regulations, applicable law, standards of professional conduct and practice, and community attitudes." This being the case, the guidelines state that "the committee *may* therefore need to include persons whose primary concerns lie in these areas rather than in the conduct of research"[52] (my emphasis).

However, from the standpoint of the control of the conduct of human experimentation, the DHEW *Institutional Guide* requirements do not differ significantly from the PHS policies that were in effect when this study was done. That is, the primary control mechanism continues to be the peer review, which takes place when a research project is *proposed*. Such elementary social control mechanisms as monitoring and sanctions are not present in an effective way. This statement needs amplification, lest it seem to overlook certain provisions of the DHEW policy.

A "continuous review" function has appeared in PHS and DHEW statements since the beginning. The July 1, 1966 PHS policy statement[53] required review committees to "maintain surveillance," in addition to the proposal review and advisory functions. The same statement required that "the institution will assure itself that its policies and the advice of its review groups are followed."[54] Nothing was specified about how this function should be performed, and the statement itself disappeared from the 1968 PHS policy booklet.[55] However, the 1969 booklet[56] made it clear that continuing review was a committee function, but it was vague about how this should be carried out or what was required. The DHEW *Institutional Guide* continues to require continuing review, calling it "essential." This document is somewhat more specific about the continuing review requirement:

> these committees may adopt a variety of continuing review mechanisms. They may involve systematic review of projects at fixed intervals, or at intervals set by the committee commensurate with the project's risk. Thus a project involving an untried procedure may initially require reconsideration as each subject completes his involvement. A highly routine project may need no more than annual review. Routine diagnostic service procedures, such as biopsy and autopsy, which contribute to research and demonstration activities generally require no more than annual review. Spot checks may be used to supplement scheduled reviews.
>
> Actual review may involve interviews with the responsible staff, or review of written reports and supporting documents.[57]

Such a continuing review seems to be directed at the question of whether a project, once begun, continues to be justified in light of the knowledge about risks and benefits that has been gained in the research up to the time of the review. It also is directed at asssuring that proper documentation is being kept; presumably, this refers to signed consent forms. The procedure seems *not* to have been designed for the purpose of assuring that the actual conduct of the research conforms to ethical standards; there is, for example, no suggestion that subjects should be interviewed to determine if they had been informed in accordance with the DHEW definition or if their participation had in any way been coerced. This study will present evidence that suggests that a continuing review of a project should examine the authenticity of consent among its subjects along with other matters that are reviewed.

Like the continuing review requirements, the enforcement and sanctions provisions of current policies are general. Chapter 1–40 in the DHEW Grants Administration Manual contains the strongest statement on this topic:

> If, in the judgment of the Secretary, an institution fails to discharge its responsibilities for the protection of the rights and welfare of the individuals in its care, whether or not DHEW funds are involved, he may question whether the institution and the individuals concerned should remain eligible to receive future DHEW funds for activities involving human subjects.[58]

Not only is the language permissive, but the enforcement is assigned to the PHS's Division of Research Grants. However, the panel appointed by

DHEW to investigate the Tuskegee Syphilis Study concluded that the "staff members of the DRG are probably the last persons to hear of any infractions once they have occurred, and then only when, as in the Tuskegee Study, they are of major proportions."[59]

The point of concern here is the weakness of the social control mechanisms under the policies that were in effect when this study was done and under the policies that now exist. The requirements that apply once a project has secured the approval of a peer review committee do not demand to be taken seriously. This is not to denigrate the basic concept of peer review in human experimentation; rather, it is to point to a serious limitation of this regulatory procedure, which has been widely hailed as an important advance. Perhaps the most important difference between the original approval of a proposed project and the continuing review of its conduct is that funding is contingent primarily at the first stage. Since money is less likely to hinge on the continuing review, a committee of busy people is likely to find insufficient time to police the conduct of its peers. This problem was recognized by the Tuskegee Syphilis Study panel:

> Institutional review committees, already overburdened by the task of examining all new research projects, are thus also responsible for re-examining from time to time all ongoing research. If something has to give first, it tends to be this assignment. Pressed for time, the review committees assume that the initial review has satisfactorily resolved all existing problems and that a cursory continuing review is sufficient.[60]

As mentioned before, one goal of this book is to assess the effectiveness of social control by peer review. The present lack of effective continuing review and enforcement mechanisms is a point to which we return.

NOTES

1. Although these cases received widespread publicity, some references may be of use to the reader. Henry K. Beecher discusses the Willowbrook hepatitis study in considerable detail in *Research and the Individual* (Boston: Little, Brown, 1970), pp. 122–127. The radiation study is described in Stuart Auerbach and Thomas O'Toole, "Pentagon Has Contract to Test Radiation on Cancer Patients," *Washington Post,* 8 Oct. 1971, p. 1. See also a follow-up story, "Radiation of Ailing Defended," *Washington Post,* 12 Oct. 1971, p. 1. Regarding the psychosurgery cases, see Jane E. Brody, "Psychosurgery Will Face Key Test in Court Today," *New York Times,* 12 March 1973, p. 1. See also, Subcommittee on Health of the Committee on Labor and Public Welfare, United States Senate, *Hearings on Quality of Health Care—Human Experimentation,* Part 2 (Washington, D.C.: GPO, 1973). The Tuskegee Syphilis Study is closely examined in the

Final Report of the Tuskegee Syphilis Study Ad Hoc Advisory Panel (Washington, D.C.:Department of Health, Education, and Welfare, 1973).

2. *Congressional Record,* September 11, 1973, pp. S 16333–S 16352.

3. Even the first title of the previously mentioned bill establishing a National Commission for the Protection of Human Subjects is directly aimed at supporting further research by establishing a National Research Service Award program to support the training of biomedical and behavioral researchers.

4. Bosio M. Giuseppe, Jacques De Senarclens, and J. J. Groen, "Human Experimentation from the Standpoint of Spiritual Leaders," and Pope Pius XII, "The Moral Limits of Medical Research and Treatment," in *Clinical Investigation in Medicine: Legal, Ethical and Moral Aspects,* Irving Ladimer and Roger Newman, eds. (Boston: Boston University Law-Medicine Research Institute, 1963), pp. 266–285.

5. Samuel E. Stumpf, "Some Moral Dimensions of Medicine," *Annals of Internal Medicine,* 64 (1966), 460–470; Hans Jonas, "Philosophical Reflections on Experimenting with Human Subjects," *Daedalus,* 98 (1969), 219–247.

6. Paul A. Freund, "Ethical Problems in Human Experimentation," *The New England Journal of Medicine,* 273 (1965), 687–692; Paul A. Freund, "Legal Frameworks for Human Experimentation," *Daedalus,* 98 (1969), 314–324; Louis L. Jaffe, "Law as a System of Social Control," *Daedalus,* 98 (1969), 406–426.

7. Talcott Parsons, "Research with Human Subjects and the Professional Complex," *Daedalus,* 98 (1969), 325–360; Margaret Mead, "Research with Human Beings; A Model Derived from Anthropological Field Practice," *Daedalus,* 98 (1969), 361–386; Bernard Barber, "Experiments with Humans," *The Public Interest,* 6 (1967), 91–102.

8. John Lear, "Do We Need New Rules for Experiments on People?" *Saturday Review,* 5 Feb. 1966, pp. 61–70; Elinor Langer, "Human Experimentation: New York Verdict Affirms the Patient's Rights," *Saturday Review,* 11 Feb. 1966, pp. 663–666.

9. Michael Shimkin, "The Problem of Experimentation on Human Beings: The Research Worker's Point of View," *Science,* 117 (1953), 205–207; Henry K. Beecher, *Experimentation in Man* (Springfield, Ill.: Thomas, 1959); Herrman Blumgart, "The Medical Framework for Viewing the Problem of Human Experimentation," *Daedalus,* 98 (1969), 248–274; Grant W. Liddle, "The Mores of Clinical Investigation," *Journal of Clinical Investigation,* 46 (1967), 1028–1030.

10. Walsh McDermott, in the *Proceedings of the Conference on the Ethical Aspects of Experimentation on Human Subjects* (Boston: American Academy of Arts and Sciences, 1968), p. 29. Subsequently referred to as *Proceedings.*

11. Guido Calabresi, in *Proceedings,* p. 19.

12. René Dubos, "Individual Morality and Statistical Morality," in *The Changing Mores of Biomedical Research,* J. Russell Elkinton, ed. Supplement 7 of *Annals of Internal Medicine,* 67 (1967), 57–60.

13. Francis D. Moore, in *Proceedings,* p. 12.

14. Bernard Barber, John J. Lally, Julia Loughlin Makarushka, and Daniel Sullivan, *Research on Human Subjects: Problems of Social Control in Medical Experimentation* (New York: Russell Sage, 1973), p. 59 ff.

15. Guido Calabresi, "Reflections on Medical Experimentation in Humans," *Daedalus,* 98 (1969), 389.

16. The most recent statement of PHS policies and requirements regarding the use of human subjects is *The Institutional Guide to DHEW Policy on Protection of Human Subjects* (DHEW Publication No. (NIH) 72–102), 1 Dec. 1972.

17. See Alexander Mitscherlich and Fred Mielke, *Doctors of Infamy: The Story of the Nazi Medical Crimes* (New York: Henry Schuman, 1949).

18. Eliot Freidson, *The Profession of Medicine* (New York: Dodd, Mead, 1970), p. 137.

19. Department of Health, Education, and Welfare, "Protection of Human Subjects: Proposed Policy," *Federal Register,* 38, No. 194 (9 October 1973), 27882–27885.

20. A rather frequently offered suggestion. See, for example, Henry K. Beecher, *Research and the Individual* (Boston: Little, Brown, 1970), p. 79.

21. These 38 codes are reprinted in Appendix A of *Research and the Individual.*

22. Reprinted in *Research and the Individual.*

23. Subcommittee on Charge III (Jay Katz, Chairman) of the Tuskegee Syphilis Study Ad Hoc Advisory Panel, *Final Report of . . .,* pp. 29–30.

24. *The Institutional Guide to DHEW Policy on Protection of Human Subjects,* p. 8. Quoted material in this and the following quotation comes from court decisions on these issues.

25. Ibid.

26. From *Slater v. Baker and Stapleton.* Quoted in Mark S. Frankel, *The Public Health Service Guidelines Governing Research Involving Human Subjects: An Analysis of the Policy-Making Process* (Washington, D.C.: George Washington University Program of Policy Studies in Science and Technology, 1972), p. 6.

27. Beecher, *Research and the Individual,* p. 226.

28. Ibid., p. 219.

29. Vikenty Veressayev, *The Memoirs of a Physician,* translated from the Russian by Simeon Linden (New York: Knopf, 1916), See particularly pp. 332–366.

30. Ibid., p. 366.

31. Jean Heller (Associated Press), "Syphilis Victims Went Untreated in Study," *The Charlotte Observer,* 26 July 1972, p. 4A. See also U.S. Department of Health, Education and Welfare, *Report of the Secretary of the Department of the Department of Health, Education, and Welfare's Tuskegee Syphilis Study Ad Hoc Advisory Panel* (Washington, D.C.: DHEW, 1973).

32. Stephen R. Graubard, "Preface to the Issue 'Ethical Aspects of Experimentation with Human Subjects'," *Daedalus,* 98 (1969), v.

33. American Medical Association, *Report of the Commission on Research* (Chicago: AMA, 1967), pp. 27–28.

34. Frankel, op. cit., p. 1.

35. P. L. 87–781, 21 U.S.C. 355.

36. Section 505(i), Federal Food, Drug, and Cosmetic Act.

37. William J. Curran, "Governmental Regulation of the Use of Human Subjects in Medical Research: The Approach of Two Federal Agencies," *Daedalus,* 98 (1969), 566.

38. Ibid.

39. A most useful discussion of the background and development of PHS policy regarding human subjects is Frankel's, *The Public Health Service Guidelines Governing Research Involving Human Subjects, op. cit.*

40. Ibid., p. 10.

41. Quoted in Ibid., p. 16.

42. This study, conducted by the Boston University Law-Medicine Research Institute, is discussed by Frankel, p. 18, and by Curran, "Governmental Regulation . . .", pp. 546–548. The Law-Medicine Research Institute study confirmed results of a more modest contemporary study by Louis G. Welt, "Reflections on the Problems of Human Experimentation," *Connecticut Medicine,* 25 (1961), 75–79.

43. For an extensive review of this case, accompanied by many original documents, see Jay Katz, ed., *Experimentation with Human Beings* (New York: Russell Sage, 1972), pp. 9–65.

44. This point is made by both Frankel (pp. 21–23) and Curran (p. 560).

45. Henry K. Beecher, "Ethics and Clinical Research," *New England Journal of Medicine,* 274 (1966), 1354–1360.

46. I am grateful to Donald Chalkley, Chief of the Institutional Relations Branch, Division of Research Grants, NIH, DHEW, for furnishing me with copies of all PHS policy statements and many supporting documents and for answering my numerous questions regarding the background and modifications of these policies since their inception.

47. Surgeon General, "Memo to Heads of Institutions Conducting Research With Public Health Service Grants," 8 Feb. 1966.

48. Ibid.

49. Ibid.

50. The substance, and even the language, of much of the DHEW *Institutional Guide* appeared earlier in 1971 in the DHEW *Grants Administration Manual's* Chapter 1-40 on "Protection of Human Subjects." Since the differences between these documents are not important for our purposes, and because the *Institutional Guide* is the most recent policy statement, references herein will be to the DHEW *Institutional Guide* (see footnote 24).

51. *Institutional Guide . . . ,* p. 7.

52. Ibid., p. 4.

53. U.S. Public Health Service, "Investigations Involving Human Subjects, including Clinical Research: Requirements for Review to Insure the Rights and Welfare of Individuals," (PPO #129, revised), July 1, 1966.

54. Ibid., p. 3.

55. This 19 page booklet, which was apparently not circulated, is entitled *Public Health Service Policy for the Protection of the Individual as a Subject of Investigation,* (PHS Publication No. 1804), March, 1968.

56. U.S. Department of Health, Education, and Welfare, *Protection of the Individual as a Research Subject: Extramural Programs* (Washington, D.C.: GPO, 1 May 1969).

57. *Institutional Guide,* pp. 8–9.

58. *Grants Administration Manual,* (1–40–50), p. 22.

59. Subcommittee on Charge III, op. cit., (See footnote 23), p. 36.

60. Ibid., p. 35.

CHAPTER TWO

SETTING AND METHODOLOGY
OF THE STUDY

The findings and conclusions in this book are largely based on the study of research subjects in two projects in a large university medical center. While I do not suggest that the institution or research projects studied were somehow "representative" of all institutions or projects, I nevertheless believe that the relationships, processes, and problems to be described are not peculiar to the projects and institution I studied. That is, the findings can be attributed to factors other than the unique characteristics of particular researchers or to unusual practices followed at a single institution. To be more specific, I believe that the relationships, processes, and problems described have their roots in such things as the structure of procedures presently regulating the conduct of research in the United States, the social definitions of the research situation that underlie those procedures, societal estimates of the relative worth of different types of people, the nature of superordinate–subordinate relations, and from other general social processes as they operate in situations in which patients are used as experimental subjects in medical research in teaching hospitals and medical centers in this country.

This is a matter about which the reader should of course draw his own conclusions. To assist in that process, I describe in some detail the institution in which the study took place, the several sources of data, and the way in which data were gathered. The two research projects that were the primary focus of the study are fully described in Chapter Four.

So as not to embarrass anyone who cooperated with my study and because assurances of anonymity were given, personal identifying characteristics have been altered throughout this book. For the same reasons, the institution in which the study was done will not be identified by name. While this in no way detracts from my primary interest in stressing the nonidiosyncratic elements of the clinical investigation process, it does necessitate a more detailed description of the institution than might be called for were it identified by name.

The study was carried out in an 850 bed hospital, which is a constituent part of the medical complex built around the "Eastern University" School of Medicine. A brief description of the hospital and the larger institution is presented here.[1] Although there are various other units, the two major elements of the medical center are the Eastern University School of Medicine and the hospital facilities.

The hospital itself is divided into the "University" division and the "Community" division, and these divisions are in separate buildings. In general, patients of private practitioners are housed in the Community division building, and patients of the medical school faculty and of the house staff are in the University division. An exception, important to this study, is that all obstetric patients are located in the Community division building, whether or not they are patients of private practitioners. Half of one floor of the Community division building contains all of the labor and delivery rooms for the medical center, and the entire floor above this one is given over to maternity cases. For the other major specialties—surgery, medicine, pediatrics—separate and parallel facilities for private and "service" patients are located in the two divisions.

The Eastern University Medical Center mixes the three familiar functions of patient care, teaching, and medical research. There is considerable overlap between these purposes (for example, treating a patient with an experimental drug), and there are potential and real conflicts between them. Most such conflicts are between patient treatment and the other two goals.

For the three major groups of physicians within the medical center—house staff, private physicians, and medical school faculty—the functions of treatment, teaching, and research have different weights. The private practitioners deal primarily with the treatment of their private patients, largely in the Community division. The house staff—almost 300 interns and residents—is largely occupied with patient care in the University division, but also takes some responsibility for private patients in the Community division. In such cases, primary responsibility for the patients usually remains with the private physician. House staff members are also involved in research, often as co-investigators with members of the medical school faculty.

The most thorough mixing of the three functions is found in the role of the physicians on the faculty of the medical school. While their formal responsibilities are largely in the areas of teaching and treatment of patients (and varying percentages of their time are given to these activities), their professional rewards and chances for advancement depend on their research activities. The result of this combination of functions can be seen in Duff and Hollingshead's discussion of the chairmen of the medical school departments (pediatrics, surgery, etc.) who are also chiefs of the corresponding services in the hospital:

> the department chairman–chief of service is caught between the avowed objective of the hospital to care for sick people and the fundamental objectives of the university to teach and do research. In the hospital the chief bears responsibility for the care of patients on his service. He is not rewarded professionally for providing a splendid service to the community's sick poor. In the university the chairman has primary responsibility for teaching medical students and carrying out research. He *is* rewarded in generous measure with salary, honor, power, and professional prestige for research and publications from his own laboratory or from the laboratories of the younger faculty members in his department.[2]

Similarly, most professional rewards for all faculty members in the medical school come from their success in research rather than from excellence in teaching students or in providing patient care. Stephen Miller, in his study of the training of the medical elite at an institution much like the Eastern University School of Medicine, makes a similar observation about the activities that are rewarded in academic medicine: "The elite segments of medicine pay continued attention to the activity which earned them prestige and permitted them to accumulate power: They must continue to conduct medical research."[3]

Clinical fellows are a fourth group of physicians in the medical center. Heavily involved in research, they generally work in a fairly narrow specialty, usually with a particular faculty member or group of faculty members. A fellow sometimes originates and pursues his own research; often he is a co-investigator with faculty members or other fellows in one or a number of projects.

It is also important to understand the *research* orientation of the institution and the formal procedures by which research is monitored. Although the medical center combines the three purposes just described, its involvement in research is particularly significant as the source of the medical school's national reputation. One administrator described Eastern as "typical of research-oriented medical schools." The training of students, for example, reflects this; a brochure prepared for incoming medical students informs them that "a larger proportion [of students] than in most schools enters careers in teaching and research . . . the goal of the [Eastern] university medical program is to enable the student to make significant contributions to his field." Extensive research activities are associated with many other institutional features. For example, Barber et al. found that the presence of a large number of researchers at an institution was associated with several characteristics. Such institutions are more likely to be "highly productive," to have a large research budget, to be either medical schools or teaching hospitals closely affiliated with medical schools, to be institutions that "strongly encourage research," to be involved in research at the "scientific frontier," and to receive a high proportion of their research funds from the Public Health Service.[4] There is no doubt that research activities have a deep and widespread impact throughout the institution, or that Eastern University medical center is the type of highly research-oriented institution that Barber et al. describe; its research facilities are extensive, and its faculty is highly productive and nationally prominent.

A statistical indicator of the institution's emphasis on research and its national significance as a research institution comes from the support its research receives from the National Institutes of Health. NIH has been estimated (in 1971) to have at least partially supported as much as 90 percent of the "best clinical research" carried out in the country in recent years.[5] In research support from that important agency, Eastern University School of Medicine is of elite status. Calculations based on fiscal year 1969 figures and published by NIH[5] indicate that Eastern University School of Medicine was well up in the top quartile of all American medical schools both in number of research grants and awards received (more than 200) and in total number of dollars awarded (more than 10 million).

In Chapter One the U.S. Public Health Service requirement of peer review of research involving human subjects was described. This function is performed by the "Clinical Research Committee" (CRC) at Eastern University. Although the structure and functioning of the CRC is closely examined in the next chapter, a few characteristics should be mentioned as I describe the setting for this study. In particular, the data to be presented later show the CRC to be both competent and rather active and thorough in comparison to most other such institutional peer review committees. My examination of a year's activities by the CRC showed that it had a direct impact on nearly three-quarters of the projects submitted to it for review. By such standards the CRC appears to have been unusually conscientious and effective in discharging its primary function of reviewing the risks and benefits, planned means of securing consent, and the precautions to be taken in proposed research involving human subjects. That this still did not assure the participation of *informed volunteers* in research is a point that will be extensively documented and analyzed later.

In summary, the institutional setting for this study is a large, research-oriented medical center in which the extensive research activities were monitored in a prior review procedure by an active and competent peer review committee.

THE DATA

This study was originally prompted by questions about how and why people become involved as subjects in medical research. Although researchers could shed some light on such questions, the responses of subjects were obviously essential. Since no central list was available of people who were acting as subjects, and since it was important to interview subjects near the time of their participation, it was not feasible to attempt to interview a random sample of subjects at Eastern University.[7] The only practical way of systematically locating subjects was through the cooperation of the researchers in whose studies they were participants. Thus, I decided to interview a sample of researchers, to solicit the cooperation of several who had large, active projects, and to interview the subjects in a few such projects.

The data were collected in three stages, each of which will be described below. First, data were collected from Clinical Research Committee (CRC) records on projects that met a number of criteria imposed by the needs of this research. Second, interviews concerning specific research studies were conducted with a small sample of investigators. Third, research subjects in two projects were interviewed. At each stage, larger amounts of data were collected about a smaller number of research projects. Since subjects were interviewed while their participation as subjects was taking place, some additional information became available through my observation of the active research projects.

Clinical Research Committee Data.   The records of the CRC provided the only available list of research projects involving human subjects. A protocol describing each proposed project was supposed to be filed by investigators for approval by the committee.[8] I am certain that some projects were conducted without the knowledge or approval of the CRC. No such project could have been directly supported by NIH or PHS because they require review committee approval before funding. However, there was no way to locate these unreviewed projects, and the possibility of gaining researcher cooperation in such projects seemed remote anyway. Thus, this study was confined to projects in which the investigator had followed CRC (and PHS) regulations at least to the extent of submitting a protocol for peer review and approval.

During the summer of 1970 I compiled a list of projects submitted to the CRC during the 1969–1970 academic year.[9] Of the 131 projects submitted to the CRC, 120 had been approved. The remainder had either been withdrawn for various reasons (including CRC objections) or were awaiting final action, usually following CRC-suggested modifications. The 120 approved projects varied widely by type of intervention (such as surgical interventions, drug studies, psychiatric studies, experimental programs for delivery of health services, epidemiological studies, and behavioral studies including my own), by amounts of risk and benefit, by degree of illness of subjects, by number of subjects involved, and by physical location of subjects (inpatients, outpatients, patients at other hospitals).

It was apparent that not all of these projects were suitable for my purposes and that some degree of uniformity needed to be introduced into the sample of projects whose principal investigators I would approach. Certain categories of projects that seemed least suitable for the study were therefore systematically eliminated from further consideration. These included projects that involved possible special problems of consent (psychiatry and pediatrics), projects that would be particularly inconvenient to study (those using patients in other hospitals, for example), and projects that seemed unlikely to shed much light on my questions because of innocuousness or small sample size. Following these criteria, 66 projects were dropped from further consideration.[10]

One problem at this stage was that the number of subjects required by or available to many types of medical research is considerably smaller than the numbers needed for a minimally reliable analysis in social research. More than half of the projects that might otherwise have been suitable were to involve fewer than 20 subjects.[11] The rate at which subjects became involved complicated the numbers problem further. Some projects that anticipated comparatively large samples were to be stretched over long periods so that weekly or monthly rates of new subjects were quite low. Some projects eventually were deemed unsuitable for my purposes when I learned from the investigator that very few subjects would be used during the 6-month period available to me for interviews.

At this point, 54 projects remained under consideration. All were in medicine, surgery, radiology, ob/gyn, or anesthesiology, and it appeared that all would involve at least a minimally significant experimental intervention in 10 or more inpatients.[12] A summary of each project was prepared, which included available data about the investigator, the number and characteristics (age, sex, illness) of anticipated subjects, a brief description of the purpose and methodology of the study, and the investigators' assessment of risks and discomfort. Also noted were any modifications in the project suggested or required by the CRC. These data provide much of the basis for Chapter Three.

A final problem with these 54 projects was that they involved only 37 different principal investigators. The range was from the 2 investigators who had four projects down to the 27 who had only one project in the sample. It was feasible to interview an investigator about only one project because of the amount of time an interview about several projects would take. After contact was made with investigators who had more than one project, a decision was made about which project would be the focus of the interview. In some cases, an investigator turned out to have only one project currently active; in other cases the most suitable project was selected on the basis of number of subjects involved and whether the reasons for their selection and agreement seemed to be apparent.

Data from Investigators. After the previously described data were assembled from CRC records and the list of projects was trimmed to 54, efforts were begun to learn more about these projects. Researchers (or, in some cases, their colleagues) were contacted by telephone in order to determine the suitability for study of projects which seemed to be only marginally suitable and projects whose protocols had been incomplete on such important points as number of subjects, and whether their projects were active and would involve at least 10 subjects in the next 6 months or so. Suitability was conceived as a function of both how apparent were the reasons subjects were selected and their reasons for consenting, and the number of subjects to be used in upcoming months. Thus, small projects were downgraded as were relatively innocuous (low risk) projects with obvious therapeutic benefits to subjects.

On the basis of this additional information, the 54 projects were divided into three groups: suitable, marginal, and unsuitable for further study. The breakdown was as follows:

Suitable	19
Marginally suitable	8
Unsuitable	27
Researchers doing more suitable projects	10
Researchers no longer on the staff	7
Project complete or inactive	7
Project being done outside hospital	3

It was decided to interview initially only those researchers with projects in the "suitable" category because of the purposes of the researcher interview. These were multipurpose interviews intended to increase my familiarity with and understanding of medical research; to provide basic background data and, if sufficient numbers of interviews could be completed, to test hypotheses concerning types of research and sources of subjects; and to locate researchers who might cooperate by allowing their research subjects to be interviewed.[13]

Fifteen of the principal investigators in the 19 most suitable projects were interviewed during the next month in the summer of 1970.[14] After these interviews were completed, I asked the investigators in the five most suitable projects if they would cooperate with my interviewing their subjects. To their great credit, all five agreed, even though the interviews were to cover topics of some sensitivity.[15]

The projects in which investigators agreed to allow interviews with subjects were: (1) an orthopaedic surgery project involving elderly subjects with hip joint problems, (2) a drug study treating very ill, mostly elderly subjects suffering from pulmonary or arterial embolism, (3) an investigation into the use of a continuous-flow centrifuge in various studies involving leukemic patients, (4) a study in which subjects having therapeutic abortions were starved for a few days prior to their abortions in order to learn of the effects on the fetus, and (5) a double-blind study of labor-inducing drugs.

Data from Research Subjects.   Although five researchers agreed to have their subjects interviewed, only subjects in the starvation-abortion study and the labor-induction study were actually studied. I confined my study to these groups for three reasons. First, interviews in these two projects began immediately and delays were encountered in the other three projects. Second, after the first few interviews it became apparent that the exact language used by subjects was of considerable interest and importance, and the time-consuming practice of recording and transcribing subject interviews was begun. (This was also a reason why no further interviews with researchers were conducted.) Finally, it became apparent that the dissimilarities among the other three projects would create substantial additional problems of description and analysis.

Subjects in the two projects studied were similar with respect to age and sex, and each project had an aspect that made it particularly valuable for study. The labor-induction study turned out to be the *largest* active project among the final 54, and the starvation-abortion study seemingly involved the *most sacrifice* (discomfort rather than risk) for the least benefit of any project.

It was decided to interview all subjects in both projects over a 6-month period;[16] the investigators estimated that this would involve about 60 labor-induction and 15 starvation-abortion subjects. This estimate turned out to be too high, particularly in the latter study. I eventually interviewed 51 of

53 subjects in the labor-induction study[17] and 7 of 9 starvation-abortion subjects[18] during this period.

An extensive description of both the labor-induction and the starvation-abortion studies is presented in Chapter Four.

NOTES

1. More details about the structure, historical development, and governance of this institution can be found in Raymond S. Duff and August B. Hollingshead, *Sickness and Society* (New York: Harper & Row, 1968), pp. 29–43.

2. Ibid., p. 45.

3. *Prescription for Leadership: Training for the Medical Elite* (Chicago: Aldine, 1970), p. 12. Many of Miller's observations about the pervasiveness of the research function at the teaching hospitals associated with Harvard also describe the situation at Eastern University Medical Center.

4. Bernard Barber, John J. Lally, Julia Loughlin Makarushka, and Daniel Sullivan, *Research On Human Subjects: Problems of Social Control in Medical Experimentation* (New York: Russell Sage, 1973), p. 19.

5. Marvin Siperstein, "The N.I.H. and U.S. Medical Schools," *Clinical Research,* 19 (1971), 251.

6. U.S. Department of Health, Education, and Welfare, *Public Health Service Grants and Awards,* (Fiscal Year 1969 Funds, Part 1, National Institutes of Health: Research), (Washington, D.C.: GPO, 1969), Table 4.

7. Such an investigation would have been most useful only if a random sample of people who refused to act as subjects was also available, which it was not. Also, interpretation of many aspects of a study of a random sample of subjects would be very difficult because of the differences in projects in which they were subjects. A random sample of 100 subjects in an institution like Eastern University Hospital might be involved in almost as many different projects. Nevertheless, the maintenance of a central registry of research subjects at institutions conducting human experimentation would make possible some very important investigation into the conduct of these activities. For example, the inclusion of such basic variables as age, sex, race, education, and income would allow one to determine if such characteristics are systematically related to risks and benefits from research. (The important evidence of Barber et al., on this particular question will be discussed in the next chapter.)

8. Although it was not a PHS requirement, Eastern School of Medicine policy at this time was that *all* projects involving human experimentation were to be submitted to peer review by the CRC, not just proposals that were going to be proposed to PHS for funding.

9. The only projects that may not have been included were a few that were submitted to the CRC during the summer when regular meetings were not held. The limitation of the sample to a single year's projects meant that some active projects were not included in the list, since an unknown number of projects approved prior to that year were still active. However, the percentage of approved projects that are active at any particular time decreases with the length of time since approval, as projects are completed. Since a great deal of work had to be done before projects could even be identified as active or

inactive (such information was not contained in CRC records), the limitation to one year's projects was imposed as a provisional restriction to be removed if a sufficient number of suitable projects so selected could not be identified and the investigators successfully approached. This did not prove to be a problem.

10. Thirteen psychiatric projects and 24 projects in pediatrics were eliminated because the consent of third parties is sometimes involved and because of potential interviewing problems. Eight projects were eliminated because they were either epidemiological, behavioral, or health care organization projects. Five projects were eliminated because they did not seem to require a serious decision by a subject; these involved such things as the donation of a blood sample, submission to an ultrasonic treatment or X ray, or the study of tissue removed for other purposes. (These latter projects seemed not to have required CRC approval at all.) Ten projects were dropped because they involved outpatients or patients at other hospitals. Six other projects were eliminated at this point because they were to involve fewer than 10 subjects.

11. The investigators in 47 of the 54 projects still under consideration at that point had furnished the CRC with their anticipated number of subjects. Even though projects with fewer than ten subjects had already been eliminated, 27 of these 47 projects expected to involve 20 or fewer subjects. Since it was not yet known how difficult it would be to secure the necessary cooperation from researchers, it seemed prudent not to reduce the pool of possible projects below the number resulting from the cutoff point of fewer than ten subjects.

12. Some projects that ultimately proved to be unsuitable because of small numbers were among this 54, because not all investigators had provided the CRC with numbers of subjects and because the rate of subject use could usually be learned only by contacting the researcher.

13. I originally hoped to interview a larger sample of researchers once I had interviews with subjects underway. However, once begun, the subject interviews proved to be very time-consuming, and plans to do a more extensive study of researchers had to be dropped for the time being.

14. Vacations and professional meetings prevented my meeting with three investigators at that time, and one investigator asked to be contacted later. These four were grouped with the investigators in the eight marginal projects to be contacted again if time allowed or circumstances required. This did not prove necessary since cooperative researchers were located among the first 15 interviewed.

15. The questionnaire I planned to use with subjects was available to these investigators, and several examined it prior to their agreement to cooperate with me.

16. This time segment was carved out of the middle of both projects; that is, both were in progress at the beginning of the interview period and both continued after.

17. The two who were not interviewed were Puerto Rican women whose command of English was as inadequate for interview purposes as my grasp of Spanish. No one refused to be interviewed in the labor-induction study.

18. Of the two not interviewed, one was considered to be too young by the principal investigator, and the other did not want to be interviewed.

CHAPTER THREE

THE IMPACT OF PEER REVIEW
ON PROPOSED RESEARCH

In 1966 the Public Health Service established its peer review requirement to protect the "rights and welfare" of human subjects in PHS-funded research. This requirement, the development of which was described in some detail in Chapter One, can legitimately be seen as ushering in a new era in human experimentation, for previously many institutions had no formal procedures to protect subjects.[1] From a broader perspective, the PHS action assumes even greater importance, for it represents an early attempt to establish a regular procedure through which science can be regulated or "edited" on the basis of "extra-scientific" considerations.[2] As such it may be a forerunner of other such procedural developments; the long-standing argument that science must be allowed to go where it will is being increasingly challenged by arguments that ethical principles and societal consequences must be integral to decisions regarding the conduct and direction of scientific research.

Since 1966 the application of peer review requirements has been considerably broadened, which further indicates the importance of this development in the regulation of medical research. Institutional committees that were originally established to review only research to be funded by PHS now commonly attempt to review all research conducted at their institution, regardless of source of funding.[3] The expansion of peer review can also be seen in its adoption in 1971 as a departmental policy by DHEW to apply to all research it funds, including social science research.[4] The peer review concept is also increasing in importance outside the research situation; the best example is perhaps the legislation requiring the establishment of "Professional Standards Review Organizations" to review the delivery of health services for which the government acts as a third party payer.[5] Yet, despite the apparent importance of the peer review concept, its actual use in human experimentation has never been evaluated in a systematic fashion, nor has the impact of this interesting form of regulation on the *actual conduct* of clinical research been examined in any detail.*

A global assessment of the peer review procedure is outside the scope of this book, which did not even begin with peer review as a primary focus of study. Nevertheless, the data available here allow us considerable insight into the operation of peer review through the examination of the functioning and effectiveness of a single such review committee. The question of the effectiveness of Eastern University's Clinical Research Committee (CRC) will be approached in two different ways. In this chapter we will examine the CRC's *impact on proposals* submitted to it for approval; the data here indicate that the review procedure *can* have an important impact at this level. Later in this book we present data bearing on the CRC's *effect on the actual conduct of research* as it involves human subjects. The impact of peer review at this latter level is of primary importance, since the ostensible purpose of the review requirement is to assure that subjects' participation in research is as safe and ethical as possible. Whether that purpose is achieved can be known only through information supplied by research *subjects*; only a subject can reveal, for example, whether he understood what he was getting involved in and whether he felt free to refuse. No data on the effectiveness of the peer review procedure at this level has heretofore been available. As will be seen, my data suggest that present procedures are seriously inadequate.

In describing the structure and functions of the Eastern University Clinical Research Committee, I am fortunate to have available for comparison the data assembled by the Barber group from their survey of peer group review in almost 300 institutions doing medical research.[6] Thus, comparisons can be made showing the extent to which the characteristics of the Eastern University CRC are typical or unusual. Comparisons of a number of structural features of the CRC with the 293 institutions in Barber's sample are summarized in Table 1.

Table 1 shows that, like most peer review committees, the CRC did not restrict its review procedure to projects being submitted to the PHS, and all

---

* PHS has never made an evaluation study. A series of site visits were made (1967–1969), but this was done to assess the acceptability of the requirements to research institutions and to see what administrative adjustments were needed. These visits had little to do with the impact or effectiveness of these committees. No report of the findings of those site visits is now available, if indeed a formal report was ever made. The only extant data on the structure and functioning of these peer review committees come from a survey by Bernard Barber's Research Group on Human Experimentation and will be cited often in this chapter.

Table 1. Comparison of Selected Characteristics of the Eastern University Clinical Research Committee with the Barber et al. 293 Institution Sample

Characteristic	Eastern University CRC	Barber et al. Survey of 293 Institutions[a]
Committee reviews all proposals, not just those being submitted to PHS for funds	Yes	85%
All projects considered by full committee; i.e., committee not specialized	Yes	68%
Committee composed of 11 or more members	Yes (11)	25%
Majority of members not tenured faculty	Yes	none
Diversity		
Includes member who is legal authority	Yes	13%
Includes member who is basic scientist (Ph.D.)	Yes	9%
Includes representative from hospital administration	Yes	60%
Includes medical student member(s)	Yes	no data
Includes nurses	No	18%
Meets more frequently than 10 times per year	Yes (twice a month)	38%
Considers an average of more than four proposals per meeting	Yes (8–10)	24%
All proposals examined by some members before meeting	Yes	75%
Adopted practice of dealing with the reservations of even a single member	Yes	91%

[a] Barber et al., *Research on Human Subjects* (New York: Russell Sage, 1973). From Chapter Nine, "Social Control: The Structures, Processes, and Efficacy of Peer Group Review."

research projects were considered by the full committee. Eastern's CRC has more members than most such bodies, and it is particularly unusual in its heavy representation of nontenured faculty. (In fact, some discontent was expressed over the belief that nontenured faculty were generally disproportionately saddled with such "unrewarding" administrative responsibilities.) An important question is whether low ranking faculty members' performance on such a committee might be affected by fear of reprisals if they were to raise problems with (or fail to approve) proposals from higher ranked faculty members. Support for this concern comes from a study of the review committee at the University of California San Francisco Medical Center, in which several reviewers admitted that they were "swayed by the academic status of the investigator."[7] A final point about the composition of Eastern's CRC was its unusually diverse membership, which included a physician who is a national authority on legal aspects of clinical investigation, a Ph.D. professor of anatomy, an administrator from the hospital, and, most unusually, two medical students, one of whom was a Jesuit priest.

The activities of the CRC provide another indicator of the magnitude of the research effort (described in Chapter Two) at Eastern. The committee met on an average of twice a month during the academic year, and considered 8 to 10 proposals at each meeting. According to the Barber group's data, relatively few of these committees have so much activity.

In considering proposed research, the committee proceeded in the following way. Copies of all proposals to be considered were circulated to committee members in the days prior to a CRC meeting. Two members were assigned responsibility for closely reviewing each proposal and for initiating discussion at the CRC's meeting. Similarly, 75 percent of the Barber group's respondents indicated that their institution's committee had at least some members examine proposals before the committee met to consider them. Barber's group used this as an indicator of a "more intensive kind of review."[8]

The rules of the CRC allowed for decisions by majority vote. (In the Barber group's sample 41 percent indicated unanimity was required and 25 percent reported that a simple majority was required). In practice, however, votes on proposals were very rare—the chairman recalled one vote in 2 years—and the CRC normally required investigators to meet the reservations of even a single member by making appropriate modifications in their proposals. In the Barber group's sample 91 percent indicated that this was how their committees operated in practice.

In the Barber group's sample 47 percent indicated the presence of a formal appeal procedure. At Eastern the CRC was the creation of a larger committee of the general faculty, and the chairman speculated to me that appeals could be taken to this larger body. Whether this constitutes a

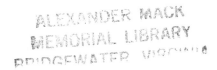

"formal procedure" as the Barber group defined it is not clear, because no such appeal had ever occurred.

The Public Health Service officially required that peer review committees "carry out interim review of the conduct of all research in such a manner and at appropriate intervals in light of apparent risks, existing administrative and supervisory organization, and other factors to assure itself that its advice is being followed."[9] However, peer review committees may be reluctant to move from the role of reviewers to the role of policemen of colleagues' performance. This is shown by the CRC's reliance solely on investigators' verbal assurances of compliance and by the fact that it had no formal provisions for continuing review other than requiring annual notices that the project was being conducted as approved. Similarly, only 36 percent of the Barber group's respondents claimed that "continuing formal review" of projects took place, and they too found indications that "continuing review" may mean very little in practice. Some of their respondents indicated that "continuing review" consisted of such things as informal discussions over lunch.[10] PHS policy statements have stressed the importance of investigators being "required" to inform their institution's review committee if changes are made in approved projects. It is probably an unusual committee for which "continuing review" means much more than such a report.

PERFORMANCE OF PEER REVIEW

More important than the formal characteristics of peer review committees and more difficult to assess is their performance. In this section, I present some data from the Eastern University CRC that bear on the committee's impact on projects submitted to it. Before presenting these data, their source—the CRC's records—should be described.

All investigators planning to do research involving human subjects were supposed to submit descriptions of their proposed projects to the CRC, using standard forms that ask for such information as the purpose of the project, the type and number of experimental subjects and controls, the duration and location of the study, and a description of the proposed methods, possible hazards, and special precautions to be taken. Also required was a copy of the proposed consent form to be signed by subjects.

Through the generous cooperation of the chairman of the CRC, I was given access to these records and to CRC correspondence with investigators. I assembled data on the actions taken by the CRC for almost a one-year period for all projects in internal medicine, surgery, ob/gyn, anesthesiology, and radiology. (Other areas, including pediatrics, psychiatry, and epidemiology were excluded for the reasons described in Chapter Two). This body of data allows us some insight into the workings of the CRC, the issues that concerned its members, and the relationship between the CRC and the clinical investigators whose proposals it judged. These investigators were of course colleagues of the members of the CRC and were in daily contact with them in other work contexts. Some proposals were from investigators who were members of the CRC; however they did not sit in judgment of their own proposals.

With regard to the impact of review committees on proposed projects submitted for review, the Barber group's study again provides some useful points of reference, although their data provide at best a crude idea* of the efficacy of these committees' performance. Their assessment of efficacy was based upon the use of four indicators: their respondents' (most of whom were members of review committees) assessments of their own committee's effectiveness, respondents' perceptions about how well their committee's work had been received within their institution, respondents' guesses about how their committee would respond to several hypothetical proposals, and respondents' estimates of the frequency with which their committee had actually rejected or required modifications in proposed research.'' There were however problems with this approach to the study of peer review efficacy. First, there turned out to be "little or no" intercorrelation among these four indicators, suggesting that a single dimension of "efficacy" was not being tapped. Second, the first three indicators were based on highly subjective judgments concerning matters about which respondents were hardly disinterested.

Only the Barber group's final indicator of efficacy—the respondents' estimates of rejection-modification rates—pertained directly to the actual performance of committees. As such these data constitute an important contribution to the question of efficacy of review. A problem with the rejection-modification data in the Barber group's study is that, in the absence of a standard against which to measure such rates, it is difficult to judge whether or not a committee is doing its job effectively. The knowledge that a committee rejects or requires modification in 10 percent of the proposals it considers does not tell us whether the committee is applying a rigorous review procedure. As the Barber group pointed out,[12] a low rate of rejection or modification could reflect laxness by a committee or it could result from a high degree of ethical soundness in proposals submitted to it. Their data give us no basis for deciding which explanation is correct. Data presented in this chapter provide a useful supplement to the Barber group's data on

---

* This crudeness was probably unavoidable in a study of a large sample of institutional review committees, which necessitated the use of mailed questionnaires, a methodology not well suited to the finer assessment of such a complex issue as efficacy.

rejection, modification, and efficacy by suggesting that it is highly probable under present conditions that a low level of rejection-modification activities by a review committee indicates that the committee is applying very lax standards.

Before moving on, we should again point out the limitations of any assessment of the impact of peer review that is based solely on the study of decision-making by the committee. Such an assessment leaves unexamined the question of whether research approved by review committees is *actually conducted* in such a way as to provide the maximum protection of subjects' health and well-being and to guarantee their rights to informed consent. This most important issue is examined later in this book. However, since the modification or rejection of even a single project (assuming proper grounds for such action were present) represents a reduction in research that either needlessly endangers subjects or inadequately protects their rights, it can be used as a measure of efficacy of review committee performance. And although this seems to be a crude indicator of efficacy, Barber's group found that it revealed a great deal of variation among institutions.

Of the institutions responding to the Barber group's survey, 34 percent reported that their review committee had *never* modified or rejected a project, a rather large number in review of the findings presented later in this chapter. The other 66 percent exhibited, in the words of Barber et al., "some degree of efficacy in improving the ethical quality of research using human subjects."[13] That is, they reported rejecting or requiring the modification of at least one project. About half of these reported having rejected at least one proposal, while the other half had required at least one revision of a proposal but had made no rejections. (In a few cases—3 percent of the committees—it was reported that while no rejections or revisions had taken place, investigators had withdrawn projects in anticipation of objections from the review committee.)

The Barber group's data on *rates* of rejection, modification, and withdrawal suggest that most committees require changes on only a small proportion of projects considered. Only 16 percent of their respondents estimated that their committees had required revision of more than 10 percent of the projects reviewed; 15 percent reported rejection rates of above 3 percent; and 9 percent estimated that more than 1 percent of projects submitted were withdrawn in anticipation of the committee's response. Only 29 percent of all the committees reported an impact higher than these levels for any of these three indicators. Thus, for the overwhelming majority of review committees surveyed by the Barber group, a direct impact on projects submitted for review was relatively unusual.

Nevertheless, 76 percent of the Barber group's respondents assessed their own review committee as being "very effective,"[14] the most positive choice available to them in a fixed-response question. This group necessarily included substantial numbers of committees that rarely rejected or modified a project, and at least 10 percent of them had to be from committees that had never modified or rejected a project or had one withdrawn in anticipation of such actions. The limitations of asking people, even professionals who are operating a self-regulation procedure, for self-assessments of the efficacy of their activities are obvious.

According to the baseline provided by Barber's data, Eastern University's Clinical Research Committee can be seen to be very conscientious and active as far as its defined responsibilities regarding proposals are concerned. During the time for which data were collected, the CRC considered 79 proposed projects from the clinical areas described above, mostly surgery, internal medicine, and ob/gyn. Of these, only 38 percent (22 projects) were approved without modification by the CRC, a very low figure in comparison to the Barber group's finding that more than one third of such committees had *never* required a modification of a project. Five submitted projects never received the approval of the CRC. It was not clear from the records what had happened in these cases, but it appeared that investigators' efforts to secure approval for these projects were dropped in the face of objections from the committee. This is not a rare occurrence according to Barber et al.[15]

The issues raised by the CRC are of some interest. They reflect the twin concerns that a research project be of sufficient promise to justify submitting subjects to its risks, and that the proposed means of securing the informed consent of subjects appear to be adequate. Thus, almost all issues raised by the CRC dealt with the design of the research, with the safety of the procedures to be followed, and with the proposed means of getting informed consent, particularly the content of the consent form itself.

The most frequently raised objections by the CRC, occurring in about two-thirds of the proposals I examined, concerned proposed consent procedures. Problems were of several types. Most commonly, the CRC felt the proposed consent form did not contain all necessary information. The importance of some of these omissions is evident in the following excerpts from CRC correspondence with investigators:

> You should mention the possibility of risk and discomfort, however minor this risk might be.

> You should mention that the drug to be used is an experimental agent. There should be some statement that use of an experimental agent entails some risk however minor this risk might be.

. . . add a statement that additional studies not directly relevant to the patient's disease are to be done before and after administration of the drug.

The consent form as it now stands does not completely describe what will be done to the patients and does not call their attention to the fact that there are risks involved in the study. It should be modified accordingly.

It should make it more clear that the patient may be receiving a placebo for as long as six months.

It should state on the consent form that an arterial catheterization will be done. It should also mention that there are some risks of both arterial catheterization and the angiographic procedure.

The consent form should indicate that _____ is an experimental preparation, and that the purpose of your studies is to demonstrate its efficacy and safety.

Closely related to the problem of omissions in proposed consent forms were instances where the CRC found that proposed consent forms were not accurate. In some cases slight but significant modification were suggested by the CRC:

Change the words "no risk" to "no known risk."

. . . in the last sentence it would be preferred if you would say that this information "may" rather than "will" help your obstetrician.

In other cases larger issues were raised, as when inconsistencies between the description of research given to the CRC differed from the description contained on the consent form. A seemingly major inconsistency is seen in the following:

It states on the consent form that no adverse effects of this drug are expected. Yet patients who take this drug by mouth have a fairly high incidence of skin rash. Also, it does not mention on the consent form the various tests you plan to do [liver and kidney function tests] as part of the study.

All told, problems of completeness or accuracy of consent forms were raised on 38 proposals, nearly half of the projects on which I collected CRC data. This was the most frequent type of problem raised by the CRC.

Because the CRC found important omissions and inaccuracies in nearly half of the consent forms they examined and required that these be corrected, it would appear that the CRC's review of proposed projects had an impact on subjects' ability to be informed before agreeing to be research subjects. Of course, this involves the assumption, which we will now examine, that researchers will comply with the peer review committee's judgments and recommendations. The CRC itself operates on this assumption, making no effort to follow up compliance (or to detect noncompliance) with their recommendations, and having no routine procedures to detect evasion of the review requirement itself. Nor are such procedures specifically required by present PHS "continuing review" regulations.

Although no systematic data concerning the validity of assumptions of good faith on the part of investigators exist, there are good reasons to doubt its universal applicability. Both Barber's group and I encountered investigators who were evading review committee procedures and requirements, a finding that suggests the need for monitoring procedures to help assure compliance by investigators. Though unsystematic, the evidence of investigator evasions of review procedures and requirements is worth citing.

One phase of the Barber group's study involved interviews with researchers at two different institutions. They were startled when 8 percent of their respondents voluntarily revealed, without even being questioned on the point, that they were conducting clinical research that had *not* gone through their institution's peer review procedure.[16] This was in direct opposition to the official policies at these two institutions.

Even though I interviewed only 15 researchers, I found similar evidence of researchers avoiding review committee requirements. Two researchers told me that they had decided not to mention their research to their subjects, even though the CRC had "required" that they secure the informed consent of subjects using written consent forms. Each of these investigators had an "explanation" for his decision to dispense with seeking the consent of subjects. One told me that his study was not of sufficient consequence to justify his spending time trying to explain it to subjects. Since his study involved no activities sufficiently unusual to alert his subjects to the experimental nature of his procedures, he was able to go ahead without mentioning anything about it to his subjects. This investigator, a postdoctoral fellow, told me that he had secured the approval of his department chairman before he dispensed with the informed consent procedure that the CRC had judged to be necessary. The other investigator was a full professor who was doing initial human trials of experimental drugs (that is, FDA Phase One investigations) on seriously ill, inoperable cancer patients. He based his decision not to inform his patients of the experimental nature of the drugs he was using on the argument that he might damage their morale by making such revelations, and that this might unfavorably affect the course of their disease. He argued that his research was therapeutic in intent and that the decision to withhold this information was within the scope of his authority as these patients' physician.*

Now the complexity of this issue is well recognized. For example, one legal authority recently commented that the physician has two separate and distinct legal obligations in such situations; one is to obtain valid consent, and the other is to act in good faith to protect the interests of the patient.[17] It has been argued that these obligations conflict in some situations. However, the fact that the issue is difficult and complex is beside the point, because it was for the very purpose of making such judgments that the peer review procedure was established. It was recognized that researchers may have strong vested interests that may interfere with their objectivity about such vital questions as whether a project is sufficiently important to justify asking subjects to take risks or whether informed consent is necessary in a particular project. It was therefore felt that such decisions were more safely left in the hands of a committee, which could perhaps examine the issues more dispassionately. Neither of these two investigators seemed to recognize that he was overruling the review committee on the very sort of decisions for which the peer review system was devised, and neither recognized the ethical problems involved in rationalizing the dispensing with informed consent in instances where it appeared that *informed* individuals *might decline* to become subjects. The fact that these two investigators, and presumably many others, could easily evade the CRC's recommendations with impunity is one consequence of the absence of monitoring procedures.

Let us further examine the types of modifications made by the CRC in research proposals submitted to it for review.

Like the first problem—incomplete or inaccurate consent forms—the second most common change required by the CRC also concerned consent forms. In 18 cases, almost one-fourth of the total, the CRC required investi-

---

* It is perhaps worth noting that the N.Y. Board of Regents, in censuring the investigators in the celebrated Brooklyn Jewish Chronic Disease Hospital case, appear to reject this argument. They held that in the experimental situation the physician has no claim to those aspects of the doctor-patient relationship that allow the withholding of information if it is deemed to be in the patient's best interests. See Elinor Langer, "Human Experimentation: New York Verdict Affirms Patient's Rights," *Science*, 151 (11 February 1966), 666. This case is described in detail in Chapter One of Jay Katz, ed., *Experimentation with Human Beings* (New York: Russell Sage, 1972).

gators to simplify the wording of their proposed consent forms:

> The consent form should be reworded in language that would be more intelligible to the average patient.

> The consent form should spell out in more detail what is to be done and why it is to be done in language intelligible to the average layman.

The CRC's instructions to investigators to simplify consent forms were stated quite similarly in all of these cases.

The CRC's concern with making consent forms intelligible to "average" persons derived from the PHS requirement that review committees assure that procedures for securing informed consent are adequate and appropriate. Although the CRC's application of its own "average person" standard resulted in its having a significant impact on proposals—almost one-fourth of the forms were rejected on this basis—there are nevertheless two important problems with its use.

First, a committee of persons with five or six or more years of training beyond college would seem to be poorly equipped to judge whether a form is written in language that the average layman can understand. Second, the concept of "average" implies the existence of a proportion (approaching 50 percent) which is less than average. (Incidently, it is not clear what dimension is involved here. That is, average with respect to what? Intelligence? Willingness to ask questions? Sophistication about medical terminology?) No code of ethics that I have seen states that informed consent is required only of the "average" subject. Even so, review committees face a practical problem in trying to find suitable language for seeking consent.* This point was made by the chairman of the CRC, who saw an early draft of this book and responded to my comment about the need to inform not only "average subjects" by saying:

> That is probably a valid suggestion. [But] at what point do we stop? What sort of form do we prepare for the individual who is

---

* The language of a consent form would matter less if such forms did not become the primary (or sole) means of communicating information to prospective subjects in some cases, as will be shown later in this book. Ideally a consent form should be accompanied by a detailed oral explanation. However, as long as there is no effective monitoring of the conduct of research, consent forms, because they are tangible, may be subjects' primary sources of information in some cases. Hence, it is appropriate for review committees to concern themselves with the language used in the forms.

totally illiterate? Et cetera. In general I feel we have to depend
upon the wishes of the investigator to proceed ethically to attempt to transmit the information we request that he put on the
form.

Except in a few situations, particularly those in which the investigator is
acting on the behalf of the subject (as when the therapy of choice happens
to be experimental), the answer would be that individuals who are not capable of giving informed consent should not be used as research subjects.
Although this is hardly a new point, the best empirical evidence available
suggests that studies with the *least favorable* ratio of risks to benefits are
the studies *most* likely to use ward or clinic patients.[18] The fact that subjects in unfavorable risk/benefit research are chosen from the segment of
the population which is, on average, least prepared to weigh the sort of
abstract information involved in informed consent does not instill confidence in the chairman's assumption that investigators will proceed ethically
to attempt to transmit the information. If that was their goal, then they
would presumably seek subjects from among the best educated and most
sophisticated segments of society rather than from among the least educated and most powerless segments. And this would be all the more so
when research involved has significant risk and little benefit for subjects.[19]

In addition to examining proposed procedures for securing consent, peer
review committees are supposed to consider the risks and benefits of
proposed research. Thus, in addition to its concerns with completeness, accuracy, and intelligibility of consent forms, the CRC also focused on the
purpose and design of proposed research. However, issues of this sort were
raised less frequently than were problems with consent forms. Nevertheless,
the CRC's actions in this area were important because they represented, in
many cases, alterations in proposed procedures for the purpose of
increasing the safety of projects. In 10 cases, 13 percent of the total, the
CRC made concrete suggestions for decreasing risks involved in a proposed
study. Such suggestions typically involved things such as closer monitoring
of subjects than had been proposed by the investigator, and the use of pre-
dictive or screening tests to try to anticipate problems or locate subjects for
which the research might be particularly unsafe. For example, in a study
proposing preoperative radiotherapy for a particular form of cancer, the
committee felt that the study should exclude subjects whose diagnosis was
doubtful in order to minimize the risks attendant to the giving of radiotherapy to those who would ultimately prove (at surgery) not to have a neo-
plasm. Here, from CRC correspondence, are other examples of the CRC's

efforts to reduce the risks or discomforts of proposed projects:

> Patients with severe post-partum pain who in the judgment of the attending obstetrician would be exposed to undue discomfort if they were to receive an ineffectual meaication must be excluded.

> As we understand it if the umbilical catheter is left in place for one hour or longer it becomes necessary to administer prophylactic antibiotics. Therefore, we request your assurance that in no case will the catheter be in place solely for purposes of study for a period of time long enough to make antibiotic administration necessary. If it is necessary to leave the catheter in place for routine diagnostic or therapeutic purposes, then, of course, it would be possible to continue studies.

> We understand that radial arterial blood samples will be studied only if puncture of that artery is required for routine diagnostic or therapeutic purposes. [That is, no permission is granted for doing that procedure solely for research purposes.]

The making of such recommendations for the purpose of increasing the safety or minimizing the risks of proposed research surely represents a key function of peer review committees. It is a function for which they should be uniquely equipped.

Incidently, the last two quotes illustrate one of the difficulties involved in effectively controlling human experimentation; they show the potential for evasion of ethical requirements if the research can be justified on therapeutic or diagnostic grounds. In each of these cases, the CRC specified the conditions under which an investigator could perform certain activities that would otherwise be prohibited. This is not to say that the CRC was trying to suggest loopholes to investigators. Such loopholes are, of course, readily apparent to investigators, and are one reason why social control efforts in this area are extremely complex and difficult.

The final major type of problem addressed by the CRC also concerned research design, but it raised issues about which the CRC seemed least certain of its mandate. A point often made in the literature on the ethics of human experimentation is that it is unethical to recruit subjects for research unless the risks to which they will be exposed are outweighed by the value of the research. Following this logic, it would be unethical to expose subjects to even minimal risk or discomfort if the research is so poorly designed as to be unlikely to produce any valid results. This would hold even if the research dealt with a topic of great importance. Thus, the CRC occasionally raised the issue of the scientific soundness of the design of proposed projects or the qualifications of investigators to do a proposed study. These issues were problematic, however, because some researchers believed that the CRC's mandate did not extend to interfering with research designs (except to reduce risk) or to judging the competence of a researcher to do what he proposed.

The CRC's willingness to raise this kind of issue can be seen in the following excerpt from a letter to an investigator from the chairman of the CRC:

> It was felt that the procedures you intend to carry out impose a considerable risk to patients who will certainly derive no benefit from them. In particular there is the need for catheterization of the bladder which has risks. To combat these risks there is also the need to administer an antibacterial drug which then imposes on the patient additional risks. There is also probably a risk of holding the administration of intravenous fluids at an absolute minimum during the procedure. Therefore, it becomes particularly important to spell out in detail what information one expects to obtain from these studies that was not available before and how the availability of this information might enhance management of similar patients in the future. In other words, is there a reasonable expectation that the information that will be obtained is worth the risk?

This line of criticism was raised only rarely by the CRC, perhaps because it tended to be resisted by investigators who may have felt that the committee had no legitimate mandate to make the judgments of competence implied by such criticisms, to say nothing of attempting to enforce such judgments by refusing to approve a project. This issue produced the most open example in the CRC's records of investigator resistance to its activities. In this case, the committee had doubts about a proposal from an obstetrician who wished to study the relative efficacy of two antidepressant drugs among patients with gynecologic malignancies who exhibited symptoms of anxiety or tension resulting from their diagnosis. At issue were his research design, which some committee members felt to be so unsound as to render his study useless, and also his competence to do psychological research, for which he had little training. The CRC encouraged him to withdraw the proposal, but he persisted. The committee ultimately yielded, perhaps because it had doubts about its authority to stop a project on any basis other than the presence of excessive risks or inadequate consent procedures.

In summary, the overall impression derived from the committee's records is that it was very active, conscientious, and effective with respect to most issues it addressed. This is not to say that the committee made all of the recommendations that it "should" have made; there is no absolute standard against which the performance of the CRC can be judged. However, using the data gathered by Barber's group as a baseline, the Eastern CRC had a high degree of efficacy in performing the function of considering proposals. It had a direct impact on nearly three-quarters of the projects submitted to it. In addition, because it was so active it may have had the further impact of causing investigators to plan projects more carefully in anticipation of the CRC's review.

Perhaps a few words should be said about my seeming assumption that a large number of changes and modifications required by the CRC were an indication of the application of fairly strict standards by a conscientious membership. Barber et al. pointed out that the taking of few actions by a committee may indicate either that it is not applying very strict standards or that few proposals with ethical deficiencies are submitted to it. In the absence of data on the reasons why peer review committees take action on proposals, Barber et al. are certainly correct in stating that there is no way of choosing between these alternatives. Data on nonactive committees might be the best for this purpose. However, the types of modifications made by the CRC suggest that the present level of consciousness of ethical issues among researchers—even among the sophisticated researchers at an institution like Eastern University is sufficiently low so as to provide ample need for review committee action. Thus, at the present time a record of few actions by a committee would seem to be a good indicator that its members are indifferent or its standards are loose. As time passes and as peer review committees educate investigators as to what will and what will not be accepted, some of the basic deficiencies in proposals will presumably decrease in frequency, and committees will need to take fewer actions. At present, however, there seems to be a need for high levels of activity and high standards of ethics on the part of review committees. Thus, the Barber group's findings on the relative lack of activity by most review committees suggest that present practices do not conform with present ethical standards.

I wish to stress again, however, that peer review effectiveness in reviewing proposals is not a guarantee that high ethical standards will prevail in actual research situations, except to the extent that committees eliminate unnecessary risks and produce corrections in unclear or incomplete consent forms. These products of the peer review system are by no means unimportant. At the same time it should be recognized that a social control system based almost entirely on reviews of *proposals* allows great opportunities for intentional or unintentional violation of such accepted precepts as the right of subjects to give informed consent. How people who did *not* give informed consent became subjects in a project that apparently conformed to review committee requirements is an aspect of the assessment presented in later chapters of the impact of current review procedures on *actual* research.

AN ALTERNATIVE VIEW OF THE PEER REVIEW REQUIREMENT

The discussion thus far has proceeded as if the peer review procedure had but one purpose—to protect the rights and welfare of human subjects. In the final section of this chapter, I want to suggest why *we should not assume that the official purpose of the peer review committees is their sole, or even primary, purpose.* We should not be too quick to accept the procedure at face value, partly as a strategy for understanding what is taking place and partly because the procedure was instituted by an agency which, as the nation's largest source of biomedical research funds, has a bias in favor of research, and because it is administered by research institutions that share this bias.

A basic fact about institutional peer review committees is that many were established so that their institutions could remain eligible to receive research funds from the Public Health Service. When an organization adopts a procedure in order to satisfy external requirements, one must be alert to the possibility that the procedure will be long on appearances and short on substance. Whether or not the procedure genuinely meets the official goal, it must *appear* to the outside audience to do so. Thus, we should carefully examine claims of successful self-regulation.

It is not my intent to issue a blanket condemnation of institutional peer review committees and the individuals who sit on them. I share the general opinion that the PHS's peer review requirements represented an important advance toward the goal of ethics in research, and I know that review committees contain individuals who have deep concerns about the ethics of human experimentation. However, we should expect great variation from committee to committee (and from member to member) in the extent to which the official goal of protecting subjects is genuinely pursued. We should also expect that in some cases the peer review procedure will serve only other functions, the most obvious of which is to *appear to meet the official goal,* thereby keeping the institution eligible for PHS research funds and above criticism.

There are, in fact, some indications that the peer review requirements were themselves established by the Public Health Service and DHEW primarily to protect those agencies from criticism rather than to protect human subjects. This interpretation of the origins of the peer review procedure was offered recently to the Senate Health Subcommittee by Jay Katz, who is perhaps the leading expert on ethical and legal aspects of human experimentation. According to Dr. Katz:

> A reading of the transcripts of the committee meetings held prior to the establishment of the current regulations [by PHS and DHEW] suggests that there was all too little concern with giving greater protection to research subjects, and much preoccupation with protecting the agencies from judicial and congressional criticism, if anything should go wrong with a research project they had funded.[20]

The fact that the PHS has never conducted a systematic evaluation of the effectiveness of its peer review requirement in achieving its official purpose of protecting subjects lends additional weight to Katz's interpretation. It is true that the PHS policy has gone through several revisions, but the changes have been primarily administrative ones made in response to complaints or suggestions from the institutions administering the policy. A series of 40 site visits were made to institutions in 1968, but this effort was directed primarily at learning whether the policy was being accepted and put into effect as it had been envisioned.[21] While such information is of obvious administrative importance, it in no way constitutes an evaluation of the impact of the policy on the conduct of research. Primarily because these site visits showed that the policy had been "addressed with seriousness," Surgeon-General Stewart characterized the policy at that time as being "successful."[22] This again leads to the question of whether the form—setting up the peer review committees—was of greater importance than the substance—protecting human subjects.

Whatever the merits of this interpretation of the establishment of the PHS's peer review requirement, the question about the purposes served by the individual institutional peer review committees remains. In reviewing the CRC's correspondence with investigators, my attention was captured by occasional statements that seemed to have nothing to do with the committee's official function of protecting subjects. In fact, this whole line of thought about the various purposes to which the review procedure could be put was prompted by the following instruction from the CRC to an investigator:

> It should not state on the consent form that medical and professional services will be provided free of charge. Of course, the patients may be told that this is the case, but if it is on the consent form it may look like coercion.

One might well ask whether something that appears to a review committee to be coercive might not be coercive to a subject, and whether it will be less coercive to a subject if it is only revealed orally.* This leads to the more basic question—for whose benefit did the CRC request this investigator to modify his consent form?

The obvious answer is that such committees have interest in protecting the institutions of which they are creatures.† Such committees may also be concerned with protecting the interests of investigators who are, after all, colleagues of the committee members. The committee may also have its own interests—at minimum, its own legitimacy—to protect. (Then there is the question of the interests of the various members of the committee, but this is leading us afield.) The suggestion that peer review committees have institutional self-protection interests should not be surprising. Many of them were created to keep their institution and its investigators eligible for PHS research funds, and the majority of such committees include among their members a representative (or representatives) of their institution's administration.[23]

Even if it is true that peer review committees serve to protect the institution that created them, it can be argued that this function may not necessarily be inconsistent with the subject protection function. Indeed, my review of CRC records located numerous recommendations to investigators that probably had the effect of protecting both the interests of the subject and the institution. For example, one investigator was told:

> The consent form . . . should not contain any statements about renouncing rights or absolving [you] from blame; such statements have no legal validity as they will not stand up in court and serve only to intimidate or antagonize patients.

The question of the extent to which such unofficial functions as institutional self-protection actually interfere with, or substitute for, the official function of peer review is an empirical question. It is not a question that I will attempt to answer here, for it requires comparative study of the activities of several committees. However, I hope to demonstrate the importance of the problem and to discuss some of its dimensions.

A hypothetical continuum along which review committees may be arrayed can be described rather easily. At one end would be committees that

---

* The question of whether such inducements are *in fact* excessively coercive is important, but is not relevant to the present discussion.

† This discussion is directed at a generic problem and is in no way intended as an indictment of the particular review committee I studied. Its performance, which has been described in detail in this chapter, suggests that its members took the subject protection responsibilities more seriously than do most such committees, using the Barber group's data as a yardstick.

exist only because they are required to exist. The fact that one-third of the institutions surveyed by Barber's group had *never* rejected or required modification of a proposal suggests that the distribution may be skewed in this direction.

Not far from this end of the continuum would be committees that are primarily concerned with maintaining the appearance of propriety. Such a committee would be more concerned with building a record (in case of future trouble) than with effectively protecting subjects, and would be satisfied if the formal requirements are met. A description of such an approach to ethical problems was offered in another context by Dr. Geoffrey Edsall. His example was not of a PHS-mandated review committee, but rather involved a World Health Organization project. Dr. Edsall recalled to the November 1967 Daedalus conference on human experimentation:

> I went to British Guiana eight years ago for the World Health Organization to see if a typhoid-vaccine study could be set up; it turned out that it could be set up very well there. I then went to London to discuss this with the people who would set such a program in motion. They asked what mechanism was going to be set up to get permission from the parents to have their children used in this study. I said that if we set up a mechanism for getting permission from parents to do the study, we would not have a study, because the parents of Guianan schoolchildren would not understand the question. The Guianans solved this problem themselves; the administrator of health set up a reverse mechanism whereby each child was given a slip to take to his parents. The children were told to have their parents sign the slip and return it if they did not want them to take part in the study. There was no trouble; the study went on for seven years before they began to run out of susceptible children.[24]

At the other end of the continuum would be review comittees that have a genuine commitment to the protection of human rights. It is worth pointing out that such commitment could be rooted in institutional self-interest as well, since doing "ethical" research is probably the most certain way of protecting the institution. However, the costs of a maximally effective peer review would be likely to appear elsewhere. Most immediately would be the costs in hostility and antagonism from researcher-colleagues whose proposals come under fire. Their reaction may be the major source of pressure on committees, creating a bias toward research.

A cost about which some concern has been expressed is that a truly effective review system might retard the development of new knowledge. Coming from researchers who, like all professionals, prize their autonomy, this argument can appear self-serving. However, it has been offered by independent observers as well,[25] and it is certainly an important concern. Although I will not try to resolve it here, I will return to it in the last chapter. However, one other aspect of the existing system of peer review suggests that there may have been some exaggeration in the fears that have been expressed about "unnecessary" restrictions upon research.

The point I wish to make is that the peer review requirement is, by its very nature, *biased in favor of doing research*. The review committees share researchers' views of the world because they are predominantly composed of researchers. This point has received relatively little attention, although there have been calls for broadening the composition of committees. (DHEW recommends, but as of this writing has not required, this step.*) It was raised, however, by two participants at the Dadealus Conference on the Ethical Aspects of Experimentation on Human Subjects in November 1967. Professor Bickel of the Yale Law School expressed reservations about the fact that the committees were largely constituted of individuals committed to furthering research.[26] However, the most interesting point was made by Dr. Walsh McDermott, whose career in medical research has been most distinguished. Referring to the peer review committees, he pointed out that:

> these juries are senior men. They got to be senior by cutting and slashing their way through the ethics of clinical investigation. They are then suddenly supposed to tell young men that they cannot do the same thing. Any reflective person finds himself in difficulty here. Medical juries are simply not the kind of instrument that a jury is in our judicial processes. They are a superficial, veneer-like approach.[27]

McDermott's characterization of the peer review procedure as superficial and veneer-like again raises the question of whether the procedure may be designed more to *appear* to deal with the problem of human experimentation than actually to come to grips with it, as Katz suggested. Thus, it may not be surprising that McDermott followed his apparently severe indictment of the procedure by concluding, "I have no objection to their being so [that is, superficial and veneer-like], as long as we do not kid

---

* Just before this manuscript went to the printer, DHEW announced new regulations that appear to require broadening of committees. The two key provisions are that "no committee shall consist entirely of persons who are officers, employees, or agents, of, or are otherwise associated with the organization, apart from their membership on the committee," and that "no committee shall consist entirely of a single professional group." Office of the Secretary, DHEW, "Protection of Human Subjects," *Federal Register* (30 May 1974), p. 18918.

ourselves into thinking they are letting the investigator off the ethical hook." In taking this position, McDermott is joining a number of other observers—almost all of whom are investigators—who have discounted the importance of establishing procedural requirements to regulate human experimentation. The answer, goes this argument, is in further developing the ethical consciousness of investigators—a matter of education.[28]

Dr. McDermott's comment suggests that another important possible consequence of the peer review procedure is that it might psychologically let investigators off of the "ethical hook."* One can imagine investigators submitting to review committees projects that they would have hesitated to undertake on their own authority, and doing so in the hope that the committee might approve the project or suggest a way that the "ethical problems" might be met. It seems conceivable that the presence of a group of peers, particularly if it acts mainly to rubber-stamp proposals, might actually embolden investigators by its willingness to support their proposals.

Evidence against the occurrence of such a consequence of peer review comes from the PHS, which released figures showing that the number of ethically-questionable research proposals that reached PHS (that is, projects that were approved by institutional review committees) decreased after the first year of the policy.[29] Nevertheless, several other bits of evidence suggest that the question is worth examining empirically.

First, the Barber group found that most review committees approve without modification virtually all projects submitted for consideration. More than 70 percent of the committees they surveyed had not required revision of more than 10 percent of proposals *or* rejected more than 3 percent of them *or* acted in a combination of these ways. This suggests that the typical review committee is doing little more than lending its support to the plans of investigators.

Second, after the PHS made the 40 site visits in 1968 to assess the acceptance of their peer review requirements, Surgeon-General Stewart summarized their findings by stating that "most of the persons interviewed felt that the policy had exerted a force toward increasing the quality of clinical research" because investigators tended to specify plans more thoroughly and because of the procedure's *"engendering in the investigator of the feeling that his colleagues supported him"*[30] (my emphasis). In view of the tendency of most committees merely to rubber-stamp investigators' plans, the engendering in investigators of such feelings as a result of the procedure

---

* Another possibility is that the peer review procedure may take some investigators off of the legal hook as well. Thus far, however, I know of no case of a researcher citing peer committee approval as a defense in a lawsuit. It seems likely that under the proper circumstances it will be so used in the future.

may have regressive consequences for the goal of protecting human subjects.

Third, there is the fact that the people most immediately affected by committee decisions are investigators, not subjects. Furthermore, an investigator can object to a committee decision, thereby prolonging its consideration of his project and fostering a spirit of compromise. Also, committee members may fear that a high level of activity on their part might threaten the committee's legitimacy among their colleagues. For example, the Barber group found a negative relationship between the level of activity of a committee and its members' perceptions of the "reception" of its work by researchers in the institution.[31] Such perceptions could result in committees seeking ways *to be of use to investigators.*

Such an impulse can be seen, for example, in CRC correspondence with investigators where there were instances in which the committee seemed to be attempting to be helpful to investigators in ways that could be readily understood. (None of these instances appeared to be threatening to the committee's official obligations towards subjects, but it has already been pointed out that the CRC was unusually active in its efforts to protect the rights and welfare of subjects.) In some cases the committee offered technical and methodological suggestions (not requirements) to investigators regarding their research. Since some members of the CRC were major authorities in their fields, and many applicants were just getting started professionally, such suggestions may have been quite helpful to investigators. Another example of CRC "helpfulness" came on a rather innocuous proposal on which the CRC volunteered the opinion that oral rather than written consent was sufficient, even though the investigator had not raised the question and had submitted a proposed written consent form. The committee informed him that he was proposing to go to greater lengths than necessary to satisfy the CRC.

SUMMARY

In this chapter we have examined the activities of one peer review committee and we have considered some of the less obvious implications of the peer review procedure. The performance of the CRC suggests that such committees can have an important impact on proposed research. The optimism that such a finding may engender must be tempered by the Barber group's findings that very few such committees are so active, and that most committees approve without modification virtually all projects submitted for consideration. It must also be qualified by the reminder that actions regarding *proposals* are quite distinct from actions that affect the *conduct* of research.

A committee composed primarily of clinical investigators is well qualified for certain aspects of the review function—for making recommendations for reducing risks and for judging whether a consent form covers all relevant aspects of a project. However, such committees seem poorly equipped for judging whether a consent form is written in language that will be meaningful to laymen. The other main judgment made by review committees, decisions concerning whether the risks of projects are outweighed by their benefits, would seem to be a decision that review committees could well share with representatives of the larger community, who may not have the same biases toward research that committee members from the institution are likely to have.

I also attempted to show that there is reason to ask if the peer review procedure may have purposes other than its official one of protecting subjects. Such committees obviously serve to add legitimization to the conduct of clinical research, and these legitimization functions could possibly become the primary function of some committees. From the standpoint of protecting subjects, we would be in worse shape if we believed in a bogus solution than if we had no solution at all; if there is a group present whose task it is to deal with the "ethical problems," then such problems can be given less attention by the rest of the members of the institution.

Finally, we pointed out that committees, particularly those that are relatively active in the pursuit of the official subject protection tasks, may receive negative feedback from their researcher-colleagues. The long-term effect of such pressures, in the absence of pressure in the opposite direction, may be a gradual loss of commitment to the goal of protecting subjects and an increasing role as a tool of institutions to protect themselves, and of researchers to increase the legitimacy of their activities.

NOTES

1. In *Research on Human Subjects* (New York: Russell Sage, 1973), Bernard Barber et al. report that 70 percent of the institutions they surveyed had a "review procedure which scrutinized the ethical aspects of proposed clinical research before the National Institutes of Health required that one be put into effect" (p. 148). Some of these review procedures were undoubtedly established in anticipation of the PHS requirements, although 36 percent had procedures as early as 1960, according to a survey by Louis Welt, "Reflections on the Problems of Human Experimentation," *Connecticut Medicine,* 25 (1961), 75–79.

2. On the notion of "editing" science, see Amitai Etzioni, *Genetic Fix* (New York: Macmillan, 1973), particularly pp. 28–40.

3. Barber et al. report that 85 percent of the institutions they surveyed subject "all clinical research" to review (*Research on Human Subjects,* p. 149).

4. *The Institutional Guide to DHEW Policy on Protection of Human Subjects* (Washington, D.C.: DHEW, 1971).

5. For one description of this development, see Claude E. Welch, "Professional Standards Review Organizations—Problems and Prospects," *New England Journal of Medicine,* 289 (9 August 1973), 291–295.

6. *Research on Human Subjects,* op. cit. See primarily Chapter Nine.

7. Kenneth L. Melmon, Michael Grossman, and R. Curtis Morris, Jr., "Emerging Assets and Liabilities of a Committee on Human Welfare and Experimentation," *New England Journal of Medicine,* 282 (19 February 1970), 427–431.

8. *Research on Human Subjects,* p. 154.

9. U.S. Public Health Service, *Protection of the Individual as a Research Subject* (Washington, D.C.: DHEW, 1 May 1969), p. 12.

10. *Research on Human Subjects,* p. 155.

11. Ibid., pp. 157–167.

12. Ibid., p. 160.

13. Ibid.

14. Ibid., p. 162

15. Ibid., p. 159.

16. Ibid., p. 167.

17. Bernard D. Hirsh, "The Medicolegal Framework for Clinical Research in Medicine," *The Annals of the New York Academy of Sciences,* 169 (January 1970), p. 310.

18. Barber et al., *Research on Human Subjects,* pp. 53–57.

19. A most elegant argument that subjects should be sought from among the "most highly motivated, the most highly educated, and the least 'captive' members of the community" is offered by the philosopher, Hans Jonas, "Philosophical Reflections on Human Experimentation," *Daedalus,* 98 (Spring 1969), 219–247.

20. *Quality of Health Care—Human Experimentation, 1973.* Hearings Before the Subcommittee on Health of the Committee on Labor and Public Welfare, United States Senate, Part 3. Testimony in this volume was given on March 7 and 8, 1973. (Washington, D.C.: GPO, 1973). The quote from Katz is on p. 1050.

21. This interpretation of the purpose of these site visits was confirmed to me in a letter in June 1973 by Dr. Donald Chalkley of the Division of Research Grants of NIH.

22. William H. Stewart, "Foreword," *Public Health Service Policy for the Protection of the Individual as a Subject of Investigation* (Washington, D.C.: DHEW, March 1968), p. vi.

23. Barber et al., *Research on Human Subjects,* p. 152.

24. *Proceedings of the Conference on the Ethical Aspects of Experimentation on Human Subjects* (November 3 and 4, 1967), (Boston: American Academy of Arts and Sciences, 1968), p. 27.

25. See for example, David Mechanic, "Risks and Benefits," a review of Barber et al. *Research on Human Subjects,* in *Science,* 181 (20 July 1973), 255–256.

26. *Proceedings . . . ,* op. cit., pp. 22 and 23.

27. *Proceedings . . . ,* pp. 28–29.

28. This argument is often made. See, for example, Jay Katz, "The Education of the Physician-Investigator," *Daedalus,* 98 (Spring 1969), 480–501. It is sometimes asserted that the protection of human subjects is *primarily* a matter of educating and selecting investigators who have the "proper" characteristics. For an interesting argument against this position, see John J. Lally and Bernard Barber, "'The Compassionate Physician': Frequency and Social Determinants of Physician-Investigator Concern for Human Subjects," *Social Forces,* 53 (December 1974).

29. "Status Report of Experience with PPO #129," Memorandum from the Office of the Associate Director for Extramural Programs, National Institutes of Health, (31 May 1968). Cited in John Fletcher, "Realities of Patient Consent in Medical Research," *The Hastings Center Studies,* 1 (1973), 48. According to the data cited therein, "problem projects" that reached NIH after passing through institutional review committees decreased from 7.4 percent of applications in June 1966 to 1.7 percent in June 1968.

30. Stewart, op. cit.

31. *Research on Human Subjects,* pp. 163-164.

CHAPTER FOUR

BECOMING INVOLVED IN RESEARCH

The next few chapters examine several important social aspects of human experimentation. The analysis and discussion is based on interviews with subjects in two medical research projects. This chapter considers how subjects come to be involved in research and how this process differs for private and clinic patients. First, however, the two projects are described in detail, since many of the findings can be understood only in light of some of the procedures that were followed.

The projects in which the respondents were participating were (*a*) a study in which women were subjected to total caloric deprivation prior to having a therapeutic abortion, and (*b*) a double-blind labor-induction investigative drug study. Unless otherwise specified, the analysis and discussion refer to the labor-induction study, since only a few subjects were involved in the starvation-abortion study. On no tabulations are data from the two projects combined. There is no systematic attempt to compare and contrast the two studies, but such comparisons are made to enrich the discussion at particular points.

THE STARVATION-ABORTION STUDY AND ITS SUBJECTS

Officially entitled "Response to Starvation in Pregnancy," this study required an 84-hour fast by pregnant women. Women awaiting abortions were selected as subjects so that the investigators could study metabolic response of the fetus to total caloric deprivation. It should be emphasized that only the fast and *not* the abortion itself was part of the study, and that a woman's having her abortion did not depend on her agreeing to participate in the study. Agreeing to participate could, however, hasten the date of admission to the hospital.

In addition to having to stay in the hospital's clinical research unit and submit to a fast, subjects also had to give a number of blood samples and collect their urine. Besides water, subjects were allowed only unsweetened tea or coffee. Before my interviews were begun, a control group of non-pregnant women (mostly dietician interns) had also fasted. All subjects interviewed in my study were part of the experimental group, and were fasting prior to a therapeutic abortion.

Subjects in the starvation-abortion study were hospitalized on a special research floor where the necessary close control of diet and the collection of waste products were routine. Although accommodations on this floor ranged from single rooms to four-bed rooms (as in the rest of the hospital), the surroundings were considerably brighter and more pleasant than in most of the hospital.

At the end of their participation in the study the subjects received the usual saline injection to start the abortion. When labor contractions began, they were taken from the research floor to have the abortion, after which they were housed on a regular (that is, nonresearch) floor. All costs resulting from the study were paid out of project funds. Otherwise, the costs for these subjects were no different from other abortion patients;[1] from the time a woman left the research floor she was responsible for the cost. The investigators' responsibility for the care of subjects was limited to the period of their actual participation, that is, during the fast and until the amniocentesis was done.

The study was directed by an assistant professor of medicine, assisted by a postdoctoral research fellow and a resident in ob/gyn. The principal investigator reported that a larger share of his time was devoted to research than to either teaching or patient care—40 percent of his time was spent on research, and the remainder split evenly between the other two functions.

Subjects in this study became involved in the following way. Prospective subjects were picked from a list of women who had been approved for abortions by a hospital committee set up for that purpose. (This was, of course, prior to the Supreme Court's landmark decision on abortion in January 1973). A woman so chosen would then be called by either the ob/gyn resident or the research fellow involved in the project. A description of the project and arrangements for participation would be made over the telephone, often during the course of several calls. The plan, according to the principal investigator, was for the woman to be given more complete information and the consent form after she came into the hospital. As will be seen, some discrepancies between this plan and actual performance took place. The principal investigator also emphasized that the telephone solicitation for participation included explicit statements to inform prospective subjects that their having an abortion was not dependent on their agreeing to participate in the study.[2] This and other statements by the principal investigator showed a considerable degree of sensitivity to the ethical aspects of his research.

Awareness of another ethical issue was expressed by the principal investigator at the time I asked if I could interview his subjects. He was concerned that although some subjects might not want to be bothered with an interview, their names would have to be revealed in order for me to determine their willingness to be interviewed. Given the sensitive and personal nature of the reason for their hospitalization, he was hesitant about this. As a way of dealing with this genuine issue, I composed a letter, addressed to his research subjects, which described my study and indicated that I would like to do an hour-long, confidential interview. The plan was for this letter to be given to each subject by one of the researchers. If a subject did not want to grant an interview, she could then refuse, and her identity would not have been revealed to me. This seemed like a good procedure, but once I had given the principal investigator copies of the letter for subjects, I heard no more about it. Although a few of the early subjects knew in advance that I was coming, none reported having been given my letter.

Seven subjects in the starvation-abortion study were interviewed. Six of these interviews were completed during the fasting period on the second and third day; the seventh was actually interrupted by the saline injection itself and had to be completed on the second day after the abortion.[3] The seven subjects were all quite willing to talk and seemed to enjoy the distraction from the discomfort of their fast. Only one subject refused to be interviewed. According to her roommate, she was unwilling to talk to anybody—to the woman who shared her room, to her mother who visited her, or to the doctors and nurses. She seemed to be greatly depressed and spent virtually all of her time watching television.

Although no systematic analysis will be undertaken using demographic characteristics of starvation-abortion subjects, the following sketch can be given. The seven subjects ranged in age from 19 to 28. Five of the women were black and Protestant; the other two were white and Roman Catholic. Two were unmarried with no children, three were unmarried or separated and had children, and two were married with children. One had a college diploma and two others had completed a year of college, two had completed high school, and two had less education. The private-clinic patient distinction did not apply among these subjects, since they were all housed in the same clinical research facility and had no contact with physicians other than the researchers.

THE LABOR-INDUCTION DRUG STUDY AND ITS SUBJECTS

The purpose of this study was to evaluate the effect of an experimental drug on "the pregnant human uterus at term, particularly in relation to [the drug's] possible role in inducing labor, and the delivery of an intact, viable fetus."[4] At its beginning, the study involved two experimental drugs and one conventional drug. The two experimental drugs, both of Phase Three FDA status, were two varieties of a more inclusive category of drugs. Shortly after interviews began, one was withdrawn by the manufacturer because it was felt that in its existing form it was losing potency on the shelf.

The project used the double-blind methodology (with one experimental and one conventional drug) in which neither investigators nor subjects knew which drug a subject was receiving. The randomly assigned drugs were given to subjects intravenously using an infusion pump. A variety of observations and measurements were made and recorded before, during, and after the procedure. Before induction, each subject's "inducibility" was rated by the investigators on a standard scale that used the factors of dilation, effacement, and consistency of the cervix, and station and position of the fetus. This rating was an important control variable in the study. In its crudest form, this variable is dichotomized between subjects who are "difficult" and those who are "inducible," a categorization used by the researchers.

Before the drug infusion began, baseline measurements were taken of maternal vital signs (temperature, pulse, respiration, blood pressure) and fetal heart rate. At regular intervals during the induction vital signs, fetal heart rate, the frequency and severity of uterine contractions, overall uterine activity, dilation, and so on were measured and recorded. Internal fetal monitoring equipment, customarily employed only when problems are anticipated, was used on subjects in this project. This resulted in some discomfort to subjects, but had the advantage of quick detection of certain kinds of fetal problems. It also provided the researchers with continuous readings of important data. Blood samples were drawn at several points, and an extensive battery of laboratory tests was done just after admission and 12 hours after delivery. Subjects were also asked to consent to having their babies observed (with X ray and blood sample from heel) for 6 hours after birth in a separate, though related study being done by a pediatrician.

The research design also specified the length of time during which efforts would be made to start labor. All infusion of drugs was to be stopped after 10 hours. Other measures could then be taken, but the subject would be regarded as a failure to induce with regard to the research. In some cases a Caesarian section might be required. More typically another attempt to induce would be made the next day, or the subject would go home the next day to return later either to be induced again (though not in the study) or in natural labor.

Both the principal investigator, an assistant professor of obstetrics and gynecology, and his co-investigator, a postdoctoral fellow in ob/gyn, were heavily involved in research, conducting other projects in addition to the one studied. The principal investigator reported that research activities consumed 80 percent of his time; teaching and patient care shared the remainder. In the labor-induction study, the day-to-day work was divided fairly evenly between the two investigators. They were assisted by two research nurses, who each devoted full time to the study, and by a secretary who kept some of the records and prepared the randomized study medications.

The large pharmaceutical company that produced the experimental drug was also deeply involved in the project. The principal investigator reported that the company had approached him about doing the study and that he and company representatives had worked out the research design cooperatively. The pharmaceutical company also had responsibility for doing much of the analysis, although laboratory work involving material subject to deterioration was done locally by the research team. Close contact was maintained between the drug company and the principal investigator.

Subjects used regular labor and delivery rooms at the hospital, although a particular delivery room was always used because the monitoring and recording equipment necessary to the study had been set up there and was immobile. Subjects also used regular accommodations for the duration of their stay in the hospital.

Shortly after a subject's admission and after the drug infusion had been started, with the permission and knowledge of the investigators and after an explanation about the purpose and length of my interview, I did a short interview with each subject; a more extensive interview was done later. The first brief interview was done in the labor room (within an hour or so after the drug infusion started) for several reasons. In order to control for the effect of the participation experience on subjects' responses (particularly if the induction failed), some responses had to be obtained at an early stage of the experience. Since subjects' final decisions to participate were often made in the labor room after admission, the labor room was the only practical place to make first contact with the subjects and to ask questions about their understanding of the research and their reasons for participating. However, since the overall interview schedule was quite long (45 minutes to an hour), it was apparent that the bulk of the interview should not be done in the labor room. Therefore, the interview was done in two sessions, with most of the questions asked after the induction was completed.

My early concern that women would not be receptive to an interview in the labor room proved to be unfounded. I also erroneously anticipated that labor contractions would greatly interfere with interviews. It turned out that some women were able to continue a response right through a contraction, although I explicitly told them that we could stop whenever they wished. Others would pause for contractions. (Since the labor of these subjects was being closely followed in the research, and since labor usually had only just begun when my interview was taking place, I was often asked by the research nurses, who left the room during the interview, to keep note of the length of and interval between subjects' contractions. Detection of contractions was usually simple. In one case, however, I finished my interview without having noticed any contractions by the subject and, when I commented on this, she told me she had had three.) In no case did subjects' contractions seriously interfere with the interview, nor, apparently, did the interview interfere with the contractions. These initial interviews lasted only 5 to 10 minutes or less, and were completed several hours before women went into the final stages of labor.

Although little difficulty was encountered in interviewing women in the early stages of labor in the labor room, it was not until the second interviews, usually done the next day, that I found much actual enthusiasm for the interview among the subjects. At that time, most women were pleased and eager to talk about their experiences of the previous day, and I was a captive listener. A few second interviews lasted close to 2 hours, although the norm was between 30 and 45 minutes.

The research staff, particularly the research nurses, the investigators' secretary, and the secretaries on the delivery floor provided me with much assistance through day-to-day cooperation. The usual pattern was for me to call the investigators' secretary late in an afternoon to inquire if a subject was scheduled for the next day. If so, I would call the delivery floor secretary between 7:30 and 8:00 in the morning to see if a subject had actually been admitted and was on the delivery floor. If so, I would come in immediately for the first interview. Here, the research nurses were particularly helpful. My interview became part of their routine so that, unless complications such as very fast labor intervened, 5 to 10 minutes were made available for me to be alone with the subject. These nurses told subjects I would be coming, explained my purpose, and introduced me to each one.

Because these interviews concerned a sensitive topic and took place at an unusual time (during early labor), perhaps I should briefly describe the explanation I gave to subjects. When I was alone with a subject, after being introduced as a sociologist by one of the research nurses, I would explain the purpose of the interview in general terms. In my first few interviews I discovered that not all subjects knew about the research of which they were a part. Thereafter, I did not state explicitly that I was interviewing research subjects, because I did not want to risk upsetting an uninformed subject during the early stages of her labor when she was already involved and committed to her course of action. I explained that I was interviewing people about their experiences in the hospital, and that one group of people being interviewed were women having their labor induced in the fashion that she (the subject) was. If a woman was aware that she was in research, she would interpret my statement to mean that I was interviewing women who were being induced in the research. If she was not aware that she was a subject, the explanation of my interview was still accurate and understandable. In addition to this explanation of my interests, I informed them that only a brief interview would take place in the labor room, and that I would like to do a second, more detailed interview lasting 45 minutes to an hour in the few days after delivery and before they were discharged.

Of the 51 subjects interviewed in the labor-induction study, 8 failed to deliver on the day of their induction. In cases in which women then stayed in the hospital either for normal delivery or for Caesarian section, the second interview was done after the baby was born. In cases where women were sent home, the interview was done before they were discharged on the morning after the failed induction. (In one case, an interview was finished in a subject's home 2 days after she was discharged). All of the subjects whose babies were born after administration of study medications were interviewed the second time before their discharge from the hospital. These interviews usually took place on the day after induction and delivery, at a time arranged with the subject.

Characteristics of the Labor-Induction Subjects.   Except for age and sex similarities, the labor-induction subjects were not a homogeneous group. The differences among them are important in explaining variations in such key matters as how they became involved, their knowledge of the research, their reasons for participating, and barriers to informed consent. (It is not possible to compare characteristics of individuals who agreed to participate with those who refused, because no potential subjects refused to participate.*)

---

* Few if any prospective subjects decided not to take part in research prior to admission to the hospital, so that such persons had *not* been selected out of the sample before my interviews. The private physician and the resident who furnished the majority of subjects in each category (private or clinic) reported to me than none of their patients had refused to take part in the re-

A distinction of fundamental importance in the labor-induction study is between the 18 women who had private physicians and the 33 women who were referred from the obstetrics clinic and were patients of the house staff. The significant representation of private patients was largely because the principal investigator had approached several private physicians about the study. His reasons for doing so probably stemmed from the project's need for relatively large numbers of subjects, and his friendly relations with these physicians, with whom he had frequent contact on the delivery floor. (Recall that the maternity facilities were the only ones shared by private and ward patients.) Ten of the 18 private patients in the study came from a single physician whose private practice was covered for him by the investigators when he vacationed.

One subject was a patient of a faculty member. Since she was referred to him by her own obstetrician for a particular reason (Rh problems), saw him on a continuing basis during her pregnancy, and had her baby delivered by him, she was classified as a private patient.

However, even though the principal investigator made specific efforts to include private patients in the study, there was still a considerable overrepresentation of clinic patients. Figures supplied to me by researchers working on utilization review in the same hospital show that the overall ratio of private to clinic obstetric inpatients for the years 1965 to 1969 was 3.1 to 1, while the 35 clinic patients (including the two Puerto Ricans not interviewed) taking part in the labor-induction study during the interviewing period outnumbered the 18 private patients by 1.9 to 1. The research subject population was clearly not representative of the whole hospital population with respect to the presence of a private physician. This, of course, is consistent with the widely-held belief that most medical research uses lower-class, clinic patients, a belief that was documented only as recently as the Barber group's study.[5]

The major demographic variables are all associated with the presence of a private physician. Table 2 shows that clinic and private patients came from very different segments of the community's social structure. While *all* of the private patients in the labor-induction study were white and married, more than half of the clinic patients were nonwhite and more than half were unmarried. Significant and important education differences were also present.

Since these variables are so highly interrelated, most of the analysis will use only the private-clinic distinction. Controlling for race will be particu-

search. Indeed, the majority of subjects did not know that research was to be involved until after they were admitted to the hospital. The resident did report that a few patients he approached, less than 10 percent declined to have labor induced at all, but that the research had no bearing on these decisions.

Table 2. **Demographic Characteristics of Subjects, by Private-Clinic Status (Labor-Induction Study)**

Characteristic	Patients of Private Physicians	Patients of House Staff	Total	
Race				
White	18	13	31	$\chi^2 = 14.81$
Black	0	19	19	$p < .001$
Total	18	32	50^a	
Marital status				
Not presently married	0	18	18	$\chi^2 = 12.88$
Presently married	18	15	33	$p < .001$
Total	18	33	51	
Education				
At least some college	13	4	17	$\chi^2 = 19.15$
High school degree	3	13	16	$p < .001$
Less than high school education	2	16	18	
Total	18	33	51	

^{a} Puerto Rican not included.

larly convenient, however, since there are no black private patients. Thus private patients can be compared to white and to black clinic patients. Marital status will be examined only where the presence of a husband would seem to be important (such as whether a subject sought advice from others). Subjects' education will also be used, particularly for analysis of degree of understanding of the research procedure.

Clinic patients were previously shown to be overrepresented in the research subject population. An overrepresentation of clinic patients would suggest that blacks were overrepresented, and this is the case. Although blacks made up 19 percent of the hospital's maternity population from 1965 to 1968, 36 percent of the labor-induction research subjects were black. However, when only clinic patients are examined, the percentage of black clinic patients in the study (54.3 percent) is quite similar to the percentage of blacks among all maternity clinic patients (56.9 percent).[6] Thus, because clinic patients were overrepresented, blacks were overrepresented.

Nor is the absence of blacks among the 18 private patients inconsistent with the total population of private maternity patients. In the years 1965–1968, the percentage of white among private maternity patients ranged from 92.9 to 94.7, with an overall average of 94 percent.

All of this indicates that the racial makeup of the research subject population was dependent upon the private-clinic makeup of the sample. To the extent that clinic patients were used, blacks were used.

All subjects interviewed were between the ages of 19 and 35, and had at least one, but no more than five children. With the exception of one Puerto Rican woman, all subjects were born in the United States, 17 in the local community.

HOW SUBJECTS BECAME INVOLVED

The way that researchers got into actual contact with subjects differed in the two projects studied. Contact with prospective subjects in the starvation-abortion study was initiated by project staff members. In the labor-induction study, however, the usual procedure was for arrangements for a woman's induction in the study to be made a few days ahead of time by her own physician (private or house staff), who would call the research staff and schedule a day for her induction. Initial selection of suitable subjects was thus in the hands of a number of different physicians, although the investigators could and occasionally did reject candidates they found unsatisfactory—either because of possible complications, violation of such control parameters as weight or number of children, or because a woman was not sufficiently "ripe" or inducible.

Once a woman's induction was scheduled, her doctor would instruct her to come to the hospital at 7:00 A.M. on the day the induction would take place. Although not all subjects were scheduled in advance, this was the usual procedure. There were two other ways in which subjects became involved. Sometimes a woman would come directly from the obstetric clinic where she had been examined by a member of the house staff. This only occurred on mornings when the research staff was available and ready but lacked a subject—a situation that often resulted from a scheduled subject's going into labor before her induction began. If there was an obstetrics clinic on such mornings, one of the research staff would telephone the clinic and ask the residents to watch for a suitable subject. Often on such occasions, a pregnant clinic patient would be sent across the street for induction in the study. Occasionally such subjects turned out not to be "ripe" enough for an elective induction, and the investigators would then send them home. The inductions of women entering the study in this way would usually begin at 10 or 11 A.M. rather than the usual 7 A.M.

The second exception to the usual procedure for entering the study happened on two occasions and involved women who were already on the delivery floor but who were not scheduled for participation in the study. In one case, a private patient was greatly disappointed by false labor and the prospect of returning home still pregnant; her physician approached the researchers to see if they could induce her, and she was accepted into the study. The other case of an already hospitalized patient occurred on a day when the staff was present but the project had no subject. The principal investigator discovered that another faculty member was in the final stages of preparation for inducing (nonresearch) a patient because of Rh and other difficulties. At the time of this discovery, the intravenous needle was already in her arm but the drug infusion had not yet begun. After her and her physician's consent, the randomized study medication was substituted for the medication already prepared for infusion, and the induction was begun.

A standard procedure was followed in obtaining subjects' consent in the labor-induction study. After a subject was admitted to the hospital and reached the labor room, she would sign the consent form given to her by one of the research nurses. After other preparations by the nurses, the principal investigator or his co-investigator would start the infusion of one of the drugs. Although a standard procedure was followed by the researchers once subjects arrived in the labor room, subjects did not arrive there with equal knowledge about what was to happen. The initial explanation was in the hands of the various private and house staff physicians who had first selected subjects for the project. Thus, how much subjects knew about the research before they were admitted to the hospital for their inductions varied greatly, and these differences had important sources and consequences.

Excluding the two women who were already in the hospital when they became involved, only 19 of 49 labor-induction subjects knew before their admission that they were to take part in a research project. Twenty-nine knew only that they were being admitted to have their labor induced (one subject's knowledge could not be assessed with certainty). However, the standard procedure followed in the labor room for obtaining consent of subjects was apparently based on the assumption that all subjects knew before admission that they were to be in research. Thus, only 9 subjects learned *in* the labor room that research was to be involved in their induction; the remaining 20 subjects learned of the research *after* the research had begun, usually during their interviews with me. All in this latter group had signed the CRC-approved consent form, but they were nevertheless unaware that *research* was involved until the interview. This seeming paradox will be explored at length in a later chapter; in this chapter our focus is on events that occurred before subjects reached the labor room and came into contact with the researchers.

Table 3 shows a difference that appears consistently in various forms throughout this study. Private patients were more likely to have had advance knowledge of the research (and to have agreed to participate before admission) than were clinic patients. It should be emphasized that we are discussing when they *learned* of the research, not when they were *told.* I have no direct knowledge of what subjects were actually told, only their *report* of what they were told. Subjects were asked to recall what they were told, and were questioned explicitly concerning the point at which they learned that research was involved. Nevertheless we must remember that we are talking about subjects' knowledge rather than physicians' behavior, although the two are obviously related.

We know, for example, that all subjects were "told" of the research in a sense, because all signed a consent form in the labor room. Nevertheless, only 9 of the 29 who did not know of the research before admission became aware of the research in the labor room. This shows the importance of the *context* in which informed consent is to take place; in this case it is apparent that the labor room was not a suitable setting for communicating information about research to prospective subjects. It also indicates that making information available is not the same thing as communicating it.

The relationship between having information available and "learning" it is fairly complex. Presumably there are many possible distinctions: what subjects are told, what it was hoped they would hear, what they heard, what they understood, what they did not want to hear, what they forgot, and

Table 3. Point at Which Subjects Learned of the Research, by Private-Clinic Status (Labor-Induction Study)

Patients	Knew of Research Before Admission	Learned of Research in Labor Room	Did Not Know of Research When Participation Began	(N)
Clinic	34% (11)	16% (5)	50% (16)	32
Private	50% (8)	25%[a] (4)	25% (4)	16

[a] Only subjects who were admitted to the hospital for the purpose of being in the study are included. Thus, the two subjects who were recruited to the project after being admitted for nonresearch purposes are not included in this cell.

what they wanted to forget. However, it is most unlikely that memory failures account for the 20 unaware subjects, because within 2 days of their inductions I asked them directly whether they had known that an experimental drug was involved in their inductions. The section on unaware subjects in Chapter Six presents several subjects responses to these questions.

The question of what information was available to prospective subjects is less important than what was *communicated* to subjects, that is, what they understood. The responsibility of securing informed consent requires investigators to *communicate,* and private patients were more likely than clinic patients to understand that they were being admitted to the hospital as research subjects. Two major variables that could explain this private-clinic difference are education and race of subjects. Although the numbers are too small to allow us to speak with great confidence, race seems the more important variable, although education also seems to have an effect.

Table 4 shows that at least 50 percent of both private and *white* clinic subjects knew of the research before admission; more clinic than private white subjects had this knowledge. Only 11 percent of black subjects possessed this knowledge on admission.

Could this racial difference among clinic patients be due to differences in education? The data show that education made no difference among private patients; 50 percent of subjects with more than high school education and 50 percent subjects with high school education or less knew of the research before admission. Similarly, half of the clinic patients who had a high school education or more were aware of the research before they were admitted. Only 19 percent of clinic patients with less than high school education had this knowledge, however.

Table 5 presents the results both by race and by education. (Because the numbers are so small, no percentages are presented.) The table shows that

Table 4. When Became Aware of Research, by Private-Clinic Status and by Race (Labor-Induction Study)

Patients	Before Admission	After Admission	(N)
White private	50% (8)	50% (8)	16
White clinic	69% (9)	31% (4)	13
Black clinic	11% (2)	89% (16)	18

Table 5. When Learned of Research: Clinic Patients, by Race and Education (Labor-Induction Study)

Subjects	Before Admission	After Admission	Total
White			
High school or more	6	1	7
Less than high school	3	3	6
Black			
High school or more	2	6	8
Less than high school	0	10	10

even among those with less than a high school education, 3 of the 6 white subjects knew of the research before admission, while none of the 10 blacks knew. Similar racial differences appear among the clinic patients with more education. It appears also that education has an effect independent of race among the clinic subjects, in contrast to the effect of education among private subjects.

The main conclusion is that information about the study was better communicated by the house staff to patients who were relatively similar to themselves with respect to race and education. (No involved house staff physician was black.) Since the labor room seems to have been a poor place to inform subjects successfully about the research, those who came into the hospital without awareness of the research were an important group.

Our focus on differences among subjects in explaining variation in their knowledge of the research should not suggest that subjects are therefore responsible for their own lack of awareness of the research. The literature on human experimentation leaves little doubt that the responsibility for communicating relevant information about research lies with the *investigator.* He is responsible for seeing that subjects understand the information that is given to them. The point is that this responsibility has been discharged more satisfactorily with some subjects than with others, and that this is related to some characteristics of subjects.

This analysis has said nothing regarding whether many subjects' lack of knowledge of the research before they were admitted was due to a failure to attempt to communicate to some patients by some physicians or whether it was due to honest but inadequate efforts to communicate with patients. I have no data on that question.

WHY PHYSICIANS INVOLVED THEIR PATIENTS IN RESEARCH

In the labor-induction study, patients became involved in the research through their physicians (house staff or private). One obvious question is why physicians involved their patients. There are important differences between private and clinic patients. This seemed to be largely a matter of whether "their" physician was acting primarily in their behalf or in behalf of the researchers. Private patients were apparently brought into the study either because of their medical needs or because they expressed great interest in being induced, and the drug study was the quickest means available. Data will be presented showing that private patients were far more likely than clinic patients to understand *why* they had been asked to participate in the labor-induction research. The existence of private patients who did not know of the research at the time they were admitted may seem somewhat inconsistent with the argument that their private physicians were acting as their agents in involving them in research. However, it is possible that some private patients were not informed about the research by their physicians because these physicians regarded the induction as a matter of treatment for the patient's benefit rather than as primarily investigative in nature.[7] In any event, there were clear indications in most cases that private physicians were acting either in the medical interest of their patients (that is, with indicated rather than elective inductions) or at their behest in involving them in the research. Also, private patients themselves seemed to see their physicians as agents to whom they could turn for advice and assurance.

In contrast to private patients, there is evidence that clinic patients were more likely to have been involved in the research because of the need for subjects rather than as a result of their own medical needs or expressed desire for induction. "Their" physicians, the house staff, seemed to be acting largely as the agents of the researchers. As was described earlier, the research staff often called the house staff on days obstetric clinics were held and asked them to find a suitable subject for the same day. Other evidence was provided by the subjects' descriptions of their knowledge of why they were asked to participate in the research, a topic we will examine in some detail.

In Miller's interesting study of interns at Harvard, an institution very similar to Eastern University in its research orientation, he used social exchange terms to describe the reasons interns furnish subjects to researchers.

> Interns obligate themselves to consulting physicians the first time
> they seek their help. In exchange for valuable information or
> services they must furnish the consultants with information

> about patients who might be useful in clinical investi-
> gation . . . When interns keep clinical investigators informed and
> permit them to use their patients, they obligate these physicians
> to provide more than information. The Thorndike [research]
> physicians recognize their obligation to interns who are sup-
> plying patients for clinical investigation. They get valuable in-
> formation from interns and reciprocate by furnishing consul-
> tation when the occasion arises.[8]

Since many interns and residents at an institution like Harvard or Eastern
have research or academic ambitions themselves, and since the sponsorship
and letters of recommendation from faculty members are essential if such
ambitions are to be realized, assistance given to clinical investigators on the
faculty also has obvious career implications.

While this social exchange formulation is useful in explaining why
interns and residents are willing to watch for patients that may be of
interest or use to clinical investigators, there are other reasons why investigators receive the cooperation from the house staff in using their patients in
research. Again, Miller points this out:

> I did not once see an intern refuse clinical investigators the per-
> mission to use his patients. An intern occasionally complained
> that the clinical investigators were using his patients as guinea
> pigs, but he knew that his complaint would not influence those in
> authority. Interns are, in fact, told that they may not always
> understand why certain procedures are necessary, or that they
> may think these things are not in the best interests of their
> patients. When they have such doubts, they are supposed to
> consult the clinical investigator. They do not need to be told that
> any difference of opinion will be resolved in favor of the latter.[9]

This is not to suggest that Eastern's house staff were unwilling adjuncts to
the labor-induction study. Acting independently, they located and made arrangements for the participation of suitable patients from the obstetrics
clinic. Since no data were collected from the house staff in my study,
Miller's findings are cited to suggest some reasons for the house staff's
willingness to assist the investigators in the labor-induction study and why
the house staff can be seen as agents of the investigators.

Subjects' Views of Why They Were Asked to Participate. There were important differences between private and clinic patients in their beliefs and
knowledge about why they were asked to participate in the labor-induction
study. To the questions, "Why were you asked to participate, do you have
any idea?" and "Why do you think *you* were asked to be a subject in this

project," (asked respectively during the first and second interviews), subjects gave four basic types of responses.

First, many subjects (almost all of whom were clinic patients) responded with the reason they were being induced rather than why they were in a research project. Typical responses were as follows:

I think because I was late and everything. (#05, white, clinic)

Because I was having a lot of trouble with the fluid and stuff.
(#09, black, clinic)

Probably because I gotta be induced. (#11, white, clinic)

I was having too much trouble. (#15, Puerto Rican, clinic)

One thing was this toxina [sic], what is it, high blood pressure.
I've had that in each one of my pregnancies, so they decided to go ahead and deliver the baby. (#18, black, clinic)

Because they said if I go too much longer I would have problems because I was gaining too much weight. (#16, white, clinic)

Well, I suppose because I was anxious to have the baby. (#43, black, clinic)

Because of the trouble I was having. (#44, black, clinic)

Because I was overdue, I guess. (#51, black, clinic)

All of these respondents gave indications that they wanted or needed to be induced, but they offered no reason why *research* was involved. Fourteen of the 48 subjects responding gave the reason they were being induced as the reason they were asked to be subjects.

The second type of response was that subjects felt they met the research criteria. Seven subjects offered this response. Some examples follow:

I fit the requirements, I guess. You know, state of pregnancy and everything. (#40, white, private)

To get my point of view, I guess. (#28, black, clinic)

I don't know. Possibly because I was overdue. I don't know. It could be any number of reasons. Possibly because I was a certain number of names down the list or something. They might have closed their eyes and just pointed [laughter]. (#30, white, clinic)

> I guess because they want to know more about it. And maybe a lot of people don't want to participate in things like that. (#31, white, private)

> I don't know. Maybe they just needed subjects. I think I was quite ready. I was dilated between three and four centimeters when I went in, so I was ready to go. And I heard Dr. M* [private physician] tell [one of the research nurses] "I told you I would send you a ripe one" so maybe they just wanted somebody that was ready or something. I really don't know. (#45, white, private)

This last subject was one of several who were not happy to be participating, a group discussed in Chapter Six.

Subjects who believed that their participation was mainly due to the researchers' need for subjects responded to this belief in two different ways. One reaction was pleasure in being able to help the researchers; subject #30 quoted above was one of the most enthusiastic participants in the study. The other reaction was an unhappy one; subject #45 quoted above felt that the needs of the research had come first and that this was not how it should have been. Which of these two reactions occurred was probably partially related to whether the subject felt free to refuse to participate. Thus, subject #45 (and we pursue this in detail later) had felt coerced; her feeling that the needs of the research were primary was translated into unhappiness at being a participant.

Some subjects seemed uncomfortable with the belief that research needs were primary, and sought reasons for their participation that gave it additional justification. Subject #24 (white, private) expressed the belief in the first interview that the needs of the research were the reasons for her participation ("[I was asked] just for the experiment, not to quicken it [her labor] because I'm basically fast"). After a successful induction, however, she gave a different reason for her participation. "At the time [I was asked to participate] I didn't know why. I figured it was that they just wanted to use me. Whereas now I know it was because I needed something to regulate my contractions and dilation so that I wouldn't dilate too fast, faster than my baby was coming." This explanation (the validity of which I cannot comment upon) was, of course, more a reason for induction than for participation in an experimental project, but it seemed to satisfy this subject, who indicated that she would be willing to do it again.

One subject in the starvation-abortion study seemed unable to accept that her participation in this study was *solely* for the benefit of the study.

---

* All doctors' initials have been changed.

Thus, she explained to me how it would benefit her, using a benefit of her own invention. A few days after she had been released from the hospital after an unsuccessful abortion attempt (which did not involve any research), she was contacted by the researchers who secured her cooperation to be hospitalized and fasted prior to another saline injection. She then decided that somehow being starved would increase the probability of success in the second abortion attempt:

> I had eaten up until I went into the hospital the other time for the injection and even that day when they called me I *was* eating, and I thought maybe that had something to do with it—why they got the blood the other time. But in the research I wouldn't eat for a few days before it. (#104)*

In response to my question, she said that the researchers had *not* told her of this "benefit."

A possible explanation for benefit invention by subjects involves the "patient role." The role of patient is a familiar one, and the role of research subject is not. One of the elements of the subject role is that the person takes a large part (informed consent) in the decision of what will be done involving him, since the physician involved has a research interest rather than, or in addition to, an interest in treating the patient. It seems possible that benefits are invented by subjects who are uncomfortable with the fact that the physician-researcher who is "treating" them may wish to subject them to a procedure for reasons that have nothing to do with judgment on his part that it will benefit them. The invented benefit makes it possible for the subject to understand the situation in terms of the familiar doctor-patient relationship. These feelings may be particularly likely to surface when patients feel that physicians, rather than themselves, are mainly responsible for making the decisions to involve them, as both of these subjects (#24 and #104) felt. Subject #24 felt she had no choice, that her private physician wanted her to be induced in the project. Subject #104 did not understand when she came to the hospital that it was for a research project; she only found this out upon admission.

The third set of reasons given by subjects to explain why they were asked to participate was that it was to their own advantage. Nine subjects gave a reason for their participation in addition to the reason they were induced and the project's need for subjects. The advantages mentioned were of two types. In a few cases medical advantages of participation were given, as with the woman who said, "my doctor felt that if the right drug was used it

---

* Labor-induction subjects are numbered 1 to 51. Starvation-abortion subjects are numbered 101 to 107.

would hasten my labor, and the baby wasn't getting any smaller" (#03, white, private). But the most frequently mentioned advantage had to do with convenience, ability to make plans, and being able to get into the hospital sooner than would have been otherwise possible, as in the following quote:

> My doctor gave us a choice. He said I could wait because I was only two or three more days, or I could come in and have it done. I guess for the very personal reason that I was getting tired of carrying myself around. It was just a matter of if I wanted to wait I could wait. So we decided to go ahead and have it. The room was available, and I was about ready to go anyway. And he gave me the option." (#22, white, private)

This third category includes only women who gave research-related benefit to themselves (medical or convenience) or to their babies as the reason why their physician had asked them to be in the research. The category does not include women who mentioned benefits that arose merely from being induced, since, presumably these benefits had nothing to do with research but only with induction. These latter women made up category one, previously described.

The fourth and largest category (18 subjects) was comprised of women who said that they did not know why they had been asked to participate. "I have no idea," (#41, white, clinic) was a typical response. Some indicated that they had welcomed being asked to participate, even though they did not know the reason for it, as in the following:

Interviewer. Why were you asked to participate, do you have any idea?

Respondent. I don't know.

I. Did you ask to be induced?

R. No, the doctor asked me.

I. Why? For what medical reason?

R. Why did he ask me? I don't know. He just asked me [said very lightly].

I. You don't know why you were asked?

R. No. I probably looked like, you know, I wanted to be or something.

I. He just out of the blue asked you if . . .

R. Yeah, he just asked me. I think he was reading my mind because I was thinking about it four weeks ago, but I didn't see [the same] doctor when I was thinking about it.

I. Were you overdue at all?

R. No. My due date is next Tuesday. [The interview was done on a Wednesday.] (#07, white, clinic)

To summarize, when questioned about why they had been asked to participate in research, subjects either indicated that they did not know, or they responded with the reason why they were induced, with the researchers' need for subjects, or with personal advantages they believed their physicians were giving them an opportunity to seize.

When patients' private or clinic status is related to these categories of beliefs about why they were asked to participate in the research, some sharp contrasts emerge that go right to the heart of the effect of private or clinic status. This is shown in Table 6.

White and black clinic patients were combined in this table because their distributions were virtually identical, and were quite different from that of the private patients. All of the nine subjects who responded that they had been asked for their own personal benefit were private patients; their physician was *their* agent. Almost half of the clinic patients did not know why they had been brought into the study, and most of the rest could only give the reason why they were induced, which indicates that they too did not know why they had been brought into the research. They only offered reasons why they had needed to be induced. These differences between private and clinic patients reflect a basic difference between private physicians and the house staff with regard to their relationships with patients.*

The house staff apparently involved their patients in the research more as a service to the researchers than because of their relationships with the

---

* A highly useful empirical analysis of the systematic differences in the hospitalization experiences of private and clinic or ward patients was carried out in this same institution by Raymond Duff and August B. Hollingshead, *Sickness and Society,* (New York: Harper & Row, 1968). Most relevant is their discussion of how physician "sponsorship" of patients varied with their social position, ranging from the "committee" sponsorship of ward patients to the "committed" sponsorship of high-status private patients. The actions of private physicians in the labor-induction study contain elements characteristic of "committed" sponsorship.

Table 6. Subjects' Perceptions of Why They Had Been Asked to Participate in the Labor-Induction Study

Patients	Personal Benefit	Needs of Research	Needed to Be Induced	Don't Know	Total	(N)
Private	52.9%	23.5%	5.9%	17.6%	100%	17
Clinic	0.0%	9.4%	43.8%	46.9%	100%	32

patients. For some of these subjects there were medical indications for induction; data furnished me by the research nurses show that 11 of the 33 clinic patients had a variety of conditions that indicated the medical need for induction of labor. The other 22, however, were elective inductions. With the exception of three subjects who recognized that they had been asked to participate because the research needed subjects, none of the remaining 19 clinic patients knew a reason for their involvement in research (though many gave me reasons why they were induced). The explanation for this must be either because they were not told the reason—if indeed their participation in the study was for their advantage—or because the primary reason for their participation was the project's need for subjects. I believe that the latter explanation is the more probable, and that house staff was acting primarily as agents of the researchers rather than of patients.

The private physicians, however, were for the most part apparently acting primarily on behalf of their patients, and were using the research for their patients' advantage. Such advantage was usually one of convenience, resulting from the fact that the research project had a labor room available to it every day, and a participant in the study could often be scheduled and admitted to the hospital more quickly than would otherwise have been possible. Medical advantages were also involved—although the experimental drug had not been proven to be superior—because of the close attention to and monitoring of subjects who were part of the study.

That the private physicians were acting as their patients' agents can be inferred from the responses of several subjects who said that it was only after they had expressed an interest in being induced or impatience with the length and discomfort of their pregnancy that they were told of the research project. By participating, they could go to the hospital either sooner or more predictably than if they waited for labor or for a nonresearch induction to be done.

The following responses indicate the private physician's role in acting on his patient's behalf in involving them in the project:

I. Why were you asked to participate?

R. Dr. D [her private physician] is a sympathetic obstetrician.

I. He knew you wanted in?

R. Yeah . . .

I. When did you first start considering being induced in the first place?

R. Uh . . . around Christmas time [two months before].

I. Really? Did Dr. D know?

R. Yes. He said under no circumstances could I have it done for convenience' sake, which at the time was primary on my mind. Not running out on my little boy at the last minute and having him all prepared. So I talked to Dr. D about it then, and got a nice healthy "We'll wait and see."

I. So your doctor knew that you wanted to be induced. Then, when did he mention that you could possibly come in this morning?

R. I think he took one look at me about two weeks ago, and I had not slept in about two weeks. I was feeling very, very wrapped up in my little self-pity and he said, "I'm not going to induce you for a while." [laughter] And I wasn't dilating as fast as I should, but he knew right then that I was ready up here [indicated her head] as soon as I was ready for it in other places.

I. When did you find that you could come in?

R. He said on Monday that it looked like I could be induced and on Tuesday he told me it would be in this program.

I. Why do you think that you were asked to be a subject in this research?

R. Because Dr. D is a friend of [the principal investigator]. (#49, white, private)

In this last statement, the subject was indicating that her physician was able to meet her desires because of his personal friendship with the principal investigator. She was very pleased that it had been possible.

Accounts from other private patients also confirmed the pattern of involvement in the research as a way of meeting the desires and wishes of the patient. Here is another example:

R. My husband is in sales. He was just recently promoted to do a lot of traveling. I became apprehensive because he was going to be gone for like 2 weeks in a row, and only home on weekends. Being new to the area—no family is around—I was getting scared. I thought, "Oh God," you know, "I hate to bother the neighbors." This type of thing. And I became very apprehensive. So at this point I had talked to Dr. D [private physician] about it and he started checking me that much sooner—having me come in on Saturdays—and said that if he thought I was prime and ready he would induce me, you know, if he thought this would be the best thing for me. So this went on for about two and a half weeks. And then when he found out when my husband would be home, then he still had me come in again and said, "Well let's see. How soon is he going out of town again?" And that's when he suggested that I come in on Wednesday.

I. Your husband was in town?

R. Right. He was in town and would be in town for another week before he had to go out of town again. So in a way it was a matter of convenience and in another way I think he might have felt I was holding back somewhat because I was frightened. And a lot of it was nerves because I was afraid I would be alone, more or less.

I. So you had a visit on Tuesday and he made arrangements for the next day.

R. Right. Right. (#36, white, private)

This private physician used the research as a way of getting his patient into the hospital faster than would otherwise have been possible, since several days notice were commonly required for an elective induction.

Similar stories of physician responsiveness were told by other subjects, all of whom were private patients:

I. How did you become involved in the research?

R. I went up on Tuesday for a regular visit and, having all of this trouble beforehand and although I wasn't late, I was getting very, very nervous and worried about the baby, and particularly since a baby did die while I was carrying it I don't think of carrying a baby as being the safest place. So I knew that once the ninth month started as far as I was concerned to have it out, whether by induction or Caesarean, was the best thing. So I was very edgy and I had counted on going home and being depressed by him saying "It's going to be another week" or whatever, because the doctor the week before [this was a three-man private practice] had said it should have been here by this time. I mean it was ready. So I joked about it and I said, "Well, Dr. R [another doctor in the group] has 24 hours to prove himself, to redeem himself or he's going to be wrong." And he said, "Well, would you like to be induced?" And I said, "You said it." And I grabbed at the chance and then he said to me—so it was after he asked me to be induced—the purpose he said is "I have a place for an inducement for, you know, educational purposes and the girl wants to be induced on Thursday rather than Wednesday. So if I can get the place, would you be interested?" And I said, "Yes." (#46, white, private)

I. Why were you asked to participate:

R. That was the only way I could get in. [pause] I feel like a ward patient or something [laughter].

I. Did you ask your doctor about being induced?

R. I had been a week overdue and I had been very uncomfortable the whole week with contractions on and off. So that I was ready and I asked him if I could go in. And he said he thought it was rather hectic, but I might be able to come in as a study patient. (#19, white, private)

Perhaps the best example of the private physician using his knowledge of the available research bed to his patient's advantage was in the case of the subject who came into the hospital in labor, but whose contractions stopped shortly thereafter. Her physician checked with the researchers, found they did not have a subject that day, and asked the woman if she wanted to participate. "He thought it was better than sending me home, because he knew I was anxious to have it" (#32, white, private). This subject was the wife of a physician who was working as a postdoctoral fellow in another part of the hospital.

The evidence presented here, of course, does not indicate that the sole reason private physicians involved some of their patients in the research was because it was a way of manipulating the hospital for the benefit of those patients. The physicians' personal and professional relationship to the researchers was undoubtedly also a factor, and there were several private patients whose knowledge of why they had been approached as subjects was as limited as that of the clinic patients. But only two of these involved elective inductions; if one applied the same argument made above concerning clinic patients, one would conclude there were strong indications that these two patients were brought into the research more as a service to the researchers than to the patients themselves. This possibility is consistent with an exchange interpretation of the friendly personal and professional relationship that existed between the researchers and the private physicians who involved patients in the study. As pointed out earlier, the practice of the physician who furnished most of the private patients in the study was covered by the researchers when he vacationed. That private physicians were to some degree acting on behalf of the researchers as well as for their patients blurs a bit the distinction made above between private physicians and house staff as acting, respectively, as agents for patients and researchers. Nevertheless, for many clinic patients, the *only* reason for their involvement in the study seems to have been the study's need for subjects; for most private patients the study was used by their physicians as a way of meeting their patients' needs, particularly as a way of getting them into the hospital sooner. No clinic patient told of such an occurrence in her relationship with the physicians of the house staff. All descriptions of verbal desires followed by physician action came from private patients. Thus, the difference between private and clinic patients remains, and is important.

Finally, let us turn to the starvation-abortion study subjects' responses to why they had been asked to participate. These subjects were perhaps more vulnerable to pressure to participate (though no evidence exists that they were intentionally pressured by the investigators), since they all reported that they had been extremely anxious to get into the hospital for their abortion at the earliest possible time. This anxiety and the feeling of vulnerability that perhaps went with it were probably responsible for the suspicion of the researchers' motives that was expressed by a few starvation-abortion subjects when I inquired as to why they had been asked to participate. Specifically, the suspicion was expressed that their anxiousness to get into the hospital had been counted on by the researchers in securing their cooperation.

This suspicion was most explicitly stated by a young black subject whose experience was as follows. After going through the hospital's procedure necessary for her to be declared eligible for an abortion, she was told that the hospital's abortion counseling office would notify her of when she could be admitted. She waited several weeks. Then one day she received a call from the researchers who told her that if she wished to take part in the starvation study, she could be admitted immediately. She agreed to do so. She then decided to check with the abortion counseling office, and learned that they had her scheduled for a regular admission the same day. Although she had been told that she would be notified by 11 A.M. on whatever day she could be admitted, the counseling office had not called her. She said of the researchers:

R. I think they just took for granted that I would come in because space was lacking. [This had been part of the reason for the delay she had experienced in being admitted to the hospital for her abortion.] Then I thought later on that they knew that I was going to be admitted that day and they got to me first before the counseling office called me. I guess they just knew that I would jump at a chance to come in because it was so late in my pregnancy. Then when I called the [abortion counseling] office—I had called them the day before and they didn't have any bed space—so I just took for granted that since they hadn't called me by 11 o'clock that day that there wasn't any bed space. I called them and checked anyway. They told me that they did have bed space. Dr. V [the resident who called her for the research project] had already talked to them, and then he had called me.

I. He talked to them?

R. Yes, She said that Dr. V called.

I. Do you know why Dr. V called?

R. No, I don't. (#102, black)

Rightly or wrongly, this subject suspected that she had been called by the researchers because they guessed how anxious she was to get into the hospital, and that they knew, but did not tell her, that she was scheduled for admission that day in any event. She honored her commitment to the researchers, however, even after she learned that she could be admitted immediately for her abortion without taking part in the research.

Two other starvation subjects may have harbored the same suspicions that their anxiety to be hospitalized had been used by the researchers, but they did not make such beliefs explicit. One said she had been asked "maybe because I was more interested in getting in and getting it over with.

So I can really enjoy my work. I was getting up against the wall, getting short-tempered. That's part of my reaction to pregnancy" (#105). Similarly, another subject said she had been asked "I think . . . because of the fact that I wanted to get this abortion over with" (#104).

The comments of two of the starvation subjects indicated that they knew they were selected because they fit the needs of the research, but evidently they saw nothing further as being involved. Subject #101 indicated she was asked "I guess because I was available; I can't think of any other reason." Similarly, subject #106 said "I think Dr. E [the principal investigator] just had a whole list of everybody, and he just hopes that somebody will agree."

Before concluding these remarks on subjects' knowledge of why they had been asked to participate in the research project, a response that was *not* given by any subjects should be mentioned. There is a belief among many minority and low-income groups that it is they who are experimented on when they come into hospitals, particularly teaching hospitals. This feeling was found by Duff and Hollingshead among their subjects,[10] and is taken as a basic assumption by the Ehrenreichs in their *American Health Empire*.[11] This same belief no doubt was behind the inclusion of a section on experimentation in a pamphlet prepared by a local, low-income neighborhood's legal-rights office. This pamphlet, "Your Rights as a Patient at [Eastern University] Hospital," was distributed to neighborhood residents who were going to be hospitalized where this research was done.

Because of these concerns and beliefs, I expected that some subjects, particularly poor or black subjects, might indicate that they had been involved in the research because they were poor, black, or clinic patients. However, no subject in either project responded in this fashion. Whether these feelings did not exist among the subjects or were present but not expressed cannot be answered.

CONCLUSION

In this chapter we have focused on subjects' reports of what took place before their active involvement in the research began, that is, before they were hospitalized. In particular, we pointed out that many subjects did not know before admission that they were to be research subjects, and that this knowledge was related to their educational level and, particularly, to their race. The actual reasons why many subjects lacked this important knowledge before admission could not be identified, since I have no data on what subjects were actually told by the various physicians who involved them in the study.

The second major point is that there were fundamental and important differences in the reasons why private and house staff physicians furnished subjects to the research. House staff members were apparently the agents of the researchers in furnishing needed subjects, while the evidence suggests that in most cases private physicians involved their patients for reasons that had to do with patients' medical needs or expressed desires to be induced as soon as possible.

NOTES

1. A cost savings for subjects was possible, however, because the time interval between the saline injection and the onset of contractions was passed on the research floor (no cost to subject) rather than on the delivery floor. It was thus possible for an occasional subject to cut a day from her time in the regular hospital facilities and, by so doing, to reduce the cost of her abortion significantly. There seemed to be little awareness of this among subjects, however, and it was not clear how often it actually occurred.

2. This description of the procedures for recruiting subjects in the starvation-abortion study was provided by the principal investigator at the time of my original interview with him, before the question of my interviewing his subjects was discussed.

3. The interviewing procedure in this study was as follows. I would call either the principal investigator's office or the research floor every few days (particularly at the beginning of the week) to find out if there was a subject. If there was, I would secure the investigator's permission and visit the subject, at which time I would either do the interview or arrange a time for it.

4. Quoted from the description of the labor-induction study submitted by the principal investigator to the Clinical Research Committee.

5. The Barber group's most important finding in this regard was that clinic patients were most likely to be used as subjects in research with unfavorable risk/benefit ratios. See *Research on Human Subjects* (New York: Russell Sage, 1973), pp. 53–57.

6. The figures for the entire maternity population of the hospital came from researchers working on hospital utilization review.

7. It was pointed out earlier that many statements of research ethics allow for lesser levels of disclosure if the intervention is undertaken to benefit the subject. It may be permissible, for example, for a doctor to withhold details of a patient's condition if he believes that such knowledge might adversely affect the patient's condition. Most of the cases in which private patients were admitted without knowledge of the research involved women for whom induction was *not* "elective." This was not the case for most clinic subjects who were admitted without this knowledge. Thus, it is possible that the reason such private patients were not informed by their physician might have been a desire not to alarm them about their condition. In the absence of data from the private physicians, however, this possibility is conjecture.

8. Stephen J. Miller, *Prescription for Leadership: Training for the Medical Elite* (Chicago: Aldine, 1970), pp. 153–154.

9. Ibid., p. 154.

10. Raymond S. Duff and August B. Hollingshead, *Sickness and Society* (New York: Harper & Row, 1968), p. 119.

11. Barbara and John Ehrenreich (Health-PAC), *The American Health Empire: Power, Profits, and Politics* (New York: Vintage, 1971).

CHAPTER FIVE

THE DECISION TO PARTICIPATE

> Any human being is more than a patient or experimental subject;
> he is a *personal* subject—every bit as much a man as the phy-
> sician-investigator. Fidelity is between man and man in these
> procedures. Consent expresses or establishes this relationship,
> and the requirement of consent sustains it.[1]

As Paul Ramsey indicates, consent is central to the ethical conduct of experimentation with human subjects. The meaning of "informed consent" is
deceptively simple: prospective subjects have a right to decide whether they
want to participate in research, and they are entitled to the information
necessary to make that decision.

The requirement of consent is not however peculiar to the research
context. It exists also in the ordinary doctor-patient relationship,* although, as Jay Katz points out, the question of what must be disclosed to
patients in therapeutic situations has never been "clearly or systematically
explored."[2] Nor is consent in either experimental or therapeutic situations
solely a matter of ethics. It has a firm legal basis:

> Anglo-American law starts with the premise of thoroughgoing
> self-determination. It follows that each man is considered to be
> master of his own body, and he may, if he be of sound mind,
> expressly prohibit the performance of life-saving surgery, or
> other medical treatment. A doctor might well believe that an
> operation or form of treatment is desirable or necessary but the
> law does not permit him to substitute his own judgment for that
> of the patient by any form of artifice or deception.[3]

---

* Consent, more generally, is basic to contract law, where fraud, misrepresentation, and
duress have long been grounds for invalidating contracts and for exacting penalties.

Such a conception of the legal base of the doctor-patient relationship is not new. For example, Judge Cardozo held in a 1914 case that "a surgeon who performs an operation without his patient's consent commits an assault, for which he is liable in damages. This is true except in cases of emergency."[4]

In recent years, as Jay Katz has written, the courts have begun to consider a patient's assent to a procedure as valid only if based upon adequate information, including risks. That is, unless one understands that to which he is agreeing, his consent is of doubtful validity. Katz notes that:

> This engrafting of the "information" component moved the concept beyond simple assault and battery law. The physician may now be held liable either for negligence in a malpractice suit, if he breaches his duty to inform a patient, or for battery, if his failure to inform is found to have vitiated the patient's consent.[5]

However, a description of this fundamental legal aspect fails to capture much that is important about the doctor-patient relationship. Even within a legal framework, the requirement of informed consent is not absolute. Relevant here are situations in which the doctor judges that certain disclosures might damage the patient's psychological state and chances of recovery, a point often made by physicians.

> Far older than the precept, "the truth, the whole truth, and nothing but the truth," is another that originates within our profession, that has always been the guide of the best physicians, and, if I may venture a prophecy, will always remain so: So far as possible, do no harm. You can do harm by the process that is quaintly called telling the truth. You can do harm by lying. In your relations with your patients you will inevitably do much harm, and this will be by no means confined to your strictly medical blunders. It will arise also from what you say and what you fail to say. But try to do as little harm as possible, not only in treatment with drugs, or with the knife, but also in treatment with words, with the expression of your sentiments and emotions. Try at all times to act upon the patient so as to modify his sentiments to his own advantage, and remember that, to this end, nothing is more effective than arousing in him the belief that you are concerned whole-heartedly and exclusively for *his* welfare.[6]

In addition to describing the most commonly cited limitation on the physician's duty to disclose, Henderson in this statement from his classic article "Physician and Patient as a Social System" exhibits a belief in the importance of a patient's *faith* in the physician. This moves us from the legal aspects to the social psychology of the doctor-patient relationship, and it is on this level that much of the analysis in this chapter will proceed.

It is essential to keep this matter of faith in mind, for it has been called the physician's most important therapeutic tool. Houston, for example, asserts:

> The great lesson . . . of medical history is that the placebo has always been the norm of medical practice, that it was only occasionally and at great intervals that anything really serviceable, such as the cure for scurvy by fresh fruits, was introduced into medical practice. By and large, the doctors were, as reported by that sane and shrewd observer, Montaigne, a danger to their patients. . . . While undoubtedly exceptional instances might be unearthed to show that these physicians accomplished something for the somatic good of their patients, in the large view we are forced to realize that their learning was a learning in how to deal with men. Their skill was a skill in dealing with the emotions of men. They themselves were the therapeutic agents by which cures were effected. Their therapeutic procedures, whether they were inert or whether they were dangerous, were placebos, symbols by which their patients' faith and their own was sustained.[7]

Since Houston wrote those words in 1938, the reality of the placebo effect has been amply demonstrated experimentally, and its therapeutic utility has come to be recognized rather than scorned.[8] Reviewing the literature on placebos, Mechanic found it to be ambiguous on many points, but it appeared that "in general, [the] placebo effects are largest when those who administer inert drugs do so with a confident sense of hope, and when those who receive them are emotionally aroused."[9]

One aspect of the doctor-patient relationship that can have dramatic consequences has been well described by Anna Freud in psychoanalytic terms:

> [The patient] comes to you with details of his life, which have really nothing to do with the doctor-patient relationship on a reality basis, and you realize that now you have ceased to be what you set out to be—the person to cure this particular individual; you have become an important person in his life, somebody who is loved, hated, on whom demands are made, from whom the patient wants interest, intimacy, preference, and suddenly you feel this must be somebody quite definite from the patient's past. He treats you as if you were his patient. *He obeys you as if you had authority over him,* or he fights against you as if he were a rebellious child. And suddenly you find that instead of having a sensible patient before you, you have become what we call an object of his transference, namely the whole load of feeling left over from earlier years—unfulfilled, disappointed— has been unloaded onto you.[10] (my emphasis)

While Anna Freud did not address the question of the physician's role in creating this situation, such a relationship between the doctor and patient has obvious implications in terms of relative power:

> I think that all doctors use the transferred positive relationships from their patients for their own advantage. *The patient is in a state of submission, admiration, obedient to the doctor.* All the better. So long as this whole trend is positive, you can use it for your own ends; you will find that your prescriptions work better, your commands are obeyed, and at least the psychological side of the patient's illness—and we know there is mostly a psychological side—will be influenced favorably. Doctors have done that always. They have done it without knowing it. It's only when this attitude becomes negative that you are in trouble.[11](my emphasis)

While not necessarily "negative," it is clear that the entry of experimental interests into the doctor-patient relationship changes the social and ethical situations. Having a subject "obey as if the doctor had authority over him" seems inconsistent with informed consent requirements of research,[12] particularly since the researcher has interests that transcend the individual subject. Thus, Capron argues that informed consent is a greater problem when an experimental intervention has therapeutic intent than in purely experimental situations:

> The "normal volunteer" solicited for an experiment is in a good position to consider the physical, psychological and monetary risks and benefits to him in consenting to participate. How much harder that is for the patient to whom an experimental technique is offered during a course of treatment. The man proposing the experiment is one to whom the patient may be deeply indebted (emotionally as well as financially) for past care and on whom he is probably dependent for his future well-being; the procedure may be offered, despite its unknown qualities, because more conventional modalities have proved ineffective. Even when a successful, but slow, recovery is being made, patients offered new therapy often have eyes only for its novelty and not for its risks.[13]

I have entered into this brief discussion of the legal aspects and social dynamics of the doctor-patient relationship because they repeatedly impinge on the experimental situation. However, the disclosure requirements in the research projects I studied did not involve a serious conflict between the researcher role and the therapist role. The disclosure and consent requirements in these projects were clear. Subjects were not being involved in research primarily for therapeutic purposes. There was no therapeutic intent in the starvation-abortion study, and while subjects in the labor-induction study stood a high chance of successfully delivering babies, conventional ways to achieve this purpose certainly existed. Furthermore, in both projects the Clinical Research Committee determined that full disclosure and informed consent were necessary.

Thus, it is clear in both projects that a researcher-subject relationship was primarily involved, although we will see that elements of the doctor-patient relationship continually intrude into the researcher-subject relationship in the medical setting. To the extent that these elements result in researcher concern for the safety of the subject, most would say it is all to the good (although it is possible to argue that an "overconcern" with subjects' welfare by researchers might inhibit the development of new knowledge). To the extent that these elements result in reduced levels of informed consent, they create ethical (and legal) problems about which much concern has been raised.

Because of the importance of informed consent in the ethics of human experimentation, the process by which subjects reach decisions and the information upon which they base these decisions are of considerable interest. These topics are the subject of this chapter; the question of *why* subjects participated in these projects is reserved for the next chapter. The findings about decision-making will not comfort those who believe that people should be subjected to experimental procedures only after they have given serious, careful thought to the matter.

THE DECISION-MAKING PROCESS

The decision process was a focal point of the interview schedule. Subjects were asked about several aspects of the decision, such as how difficult the decision was, how quickly it was made, and whether advice was sought. These questions, however, contained the unrecognized assumption that subjects were in fact making decisions. After the first few interviews it became apparent that many labor-induction subjects had not made a decision to be in research because they did not understand that research was involved. Others, who did understand that research was involved, nevertheless seemed to have given no real thought or consideration to a decision to participate. Thus, great care had to be taken to separate responses regarding the decision to have labor induced (the only decision made by subjects who were unaware of the research aspect) from responses pertaining to the decision to take part in research. In some cases it was not possible to separate these decisions, since most subjects were not presented with an alternative of having their labor induced without taking part in the study. That is, for most subjects the decision to have labor induced *was* the decision to allow possible use of an experimental drug. This was the case even though many subjects' inductions were not elective and despite the fact that nonexperimental labor inductions are commonplace.

In this section we will *not* discuss the 20 labor-induction subjects who first became aware of the research when they were interviewed after the drug infusion for their induction had begun. There is obviously no point in discussing the decision-making process for such subjects, although their existence was a most important unanticipated finding of this study; how and why so many subjects could unknowingly participate in research will later be examined in detail. *This analysis of subjects' decision-making process focuses on the 31 labor-induction study subjects who signed consent forms knowing that this meant that they would participate in a medical research project.*

For most of these subjects, the decision to receive an experimental drug was made quite lightly. Subjects were asked four questions concerning ease or difficulty of their decisions to participate in research. The items and the frequency of responses from subjects who were aware of the labor-induction research appear in Table 7. The four items approached the ease or difficulty of the decision in different ways, but the responses to all four show that subjects' decisions were usually made without hesitation or consideration of refusing.

On the last lines of Table 7, the responses to the four items are grouped into a single measure; the 55 percent who showed *no* hesitation or difficulty on *any* of the four items are separated from the remainder of the subjects. Some of the analysis will use this dichotomous grouping. The grouping procedure at the bottom of Table 7 tends to magnify the amount of difficulty subjects had with their decisions and the extent to which subjects made serious decisions. Some of the subjects who are included as "giving evidence of decision difficulty" actually reported little difficulty with the decision and answered only one item with a response that was coded as reflecting decision difficulty. For example:

I.   Did it occur to you to say no?

R.   I guess that thought ran through my mind, but at that point I just wanted to get it over with. (#27, white, private)

This response was coded that the subject *did* think of saying no. However, her other responses were that the decision was "not at all difficult," that

Table 7. Responses to Decision-Difficulty Items (Labor-Induction Study)[a]

Item[b]	Number of Subjects (31)	Percent Giving Each Response
How difficult would you say the decision was on whether or not to participate? Would you say the decision was:		
not at all difficult	25	81
somewhat difficult	6	19
very difficult	0	—
When you were asked to participate—did it occur to you to say no?		
yes	8	26
no	23	74
Did you give serious thought to refusing?		
yes	6	19
no	25	81
How much thought did you give to the decision—did you make up your mind immediately, or did you give it *some* thought, or a *great deal* of thought?		
agreed immediately	19	61
gave it some thought	8	26
great deal of thought	4	13
Subjects giving evidence of decision difficulty on at least one item	14	45
Subjects giving no evidence of decision difficulty on *any* item	17	55

[a] Only subjects who were aware of the research when their involvement began are included.

[b] The items are given as they were read to subjects. See Appendix B, items 67, 69, 70, 71.

she "did not seriously consider refusing," and that she "agreed immediately." Another interview provides a similar example:

I. Did you make up your mind immediately, or did you give it some thought or a great deal of thought?

R. I didn't really give it a great deal of thought. I would rather get it over with. (#09, black, clinic)

This subject settled on "some thought" for her answer. She showed no decision difficulty on the other three items, but she became one who "gave evidence of decision difficulty" in our coding.

Therefore, the statement that 17 of 31 subjects "gave no evidence of decision difficulty" is a conservative one. Of the 14 who expressed difficulty, 7 did so on only one of the four items—5 of them on the item on the amount of thought given to the decision. The remaining 7 expressed difficulty on three or four items.

So while some subjects gave indications of a serious decision, the majority (17 of 31) gave no evidence of hesitation or decision on *any* of the four items. Furthermore, *no one* said the decision to participate in the labor-induction study was "very difficult," only 4 subjects gave it a "great deal of thought," and only 6 gave "serious thought to refusing."

How could so many women have had no problem making the decision to allow an experimental drug to be used for a matter as important as induction of their labor? The explanation involves both the social background characteristics of the subjects and situational factors in the research setting. Data were collected on both background and situational factors, and some differences emerge, although numbers are too small to allow for detailed anlaysis of the relative importance of various factors.

Table 8 shows education and private-clinic differences concerning how serious subjects' participation decisions were. Some consistent differences among educational groups can be seen, but the same is not true of the private-clinic distinction. It appears that how seriously the decision was taken was more a function of the subjects' education than whether they had a private physician. When educational level and private-clinic status are examined together, the two largest categories—private patients with at least some college, and clinic patients with high school degrees—were quite similar on the decision difficulty variables. Six of the 11 private patients with college reported at least some difficulty with the decision; 6 of the 10 clinic patients with a high school degree reported some difficulty. (When the two clinic patients with some college are included, the figure becomes 7 of 12). However, none of the three private patients who had not attended college reported any difficulty with the decision of any of the four items; only one of the five clinic patients with less than high school education reported any difficulty. Though there are too few cases to allow a strong statement, both private and clinic patients with less education than typical for their category seemed likely to have no difficulty with their "decision" to allow the use of an experimental drug to induce their labor.

A number of situational factors were also involved in the ease with which most subjects made their decision. Some subjects offered explanations of why they had no difficulty with the decision or why they had not hesitated

Table 8. Percentage of Subjects, by Educational and Private-Clinic Status, Indicating No Difficulty in Deciding to Participate in the Labor-Induction Study[a]

Response	At Least Some College	High School Degree	Less Than High School	Private Patients	Clinic Patients
Decision was not at all difficult	69%	92%	83%	79%	82%
Did not occur to her to say no	54%	92%	83%	62%	82%
Did not seriously consider refusing	62%	92%	100%	71%	88%
Made up mind immediately	62%	50%	83%	71%	53%
No hesitation on any of items	46%	50%	83%	71%	53%
(N)	13	12	6	14	17

[a] Only subjects who were aware of the research when their involvement began are included.

to participate. These subjects often emphasized their eagerness to have their baby; many said that the *only* thing they considered was that the research might hasten this event. *The implicit choice available to most subjects was either to be induced in the research project or to wait for normal labor to begin.* Hence, such comments as the following:

R. I didn't really give it a great deal of thought. I would rather get it over with. (#09, black, clinic)

I. Did it occur to you to say no?

R. No. The only thing I think is that I am going to deliver my kid and Sunday I'll be at home. I don't care [how it's done]. (#15, Puerto Rican, clinic)

The husband of this Puerto Rican woman shed some additional light on the decision process as he translated another of her statements and offered an additional comment on his own.

R. She just signed, so it [the decision] was not difficult at all. In that
   moment maybe she was anxious about the delivery and all this, and
   she didn't care too much what was happening in terms of the experiment. I think that maybe in an unconscious way, maybe because
   we are students almost all our life, we have a bias in favor of this type
   of experiments. (Husband of #15, Puerto Rican, clinic)

Working in conjunction with their eagerness to have their baby was
considerable faith in their physicians, a factor mentioned by serveral subjects in explaining why they had no difficulty in deciding to participate. For
example, subject #48 said the decision was not at all difficult because her
doctor "said it would be easier." That was sufficient for her, and she
agreed immediately. Faith was also mentioned in the following:

R. I didn't even stop and think about refusing . . . as long as Dr. D
   [private physician] said it's all right, I went right along with him. (#12,
   white, private)

I. Did it occur to you to say no?

R. No, because I figure the doctor knows best. (#20, black, clinic)

R. I really based it on the fact that Dr. D [private physician] recommended it. Because I'm sure . . . I have absolute faith in his judgment,
   and I figure that he wouldn't recommend something that he felt would
   be harmful. I should put it that way. (#32, white, private)

I. Did it occur to you to say no?

R. No, because as I say, if my doctor says "Well, I feel this is what you
   should do," I would have done it, you know, without doubt if that's
   what he told me to do. I mean, any person not being a doctor would
   feel the same way. If they are going to a specialist and he says, "Well,
   take this vitamin," you take it. (#29, white, private)

These statements are remarkable testimony to the extent to which some
patients place faith and trust in their physicians. These women are saying
that a simple statement from their doctor made nonproblematic their decisions to allow an experimental drug to be used to induce their labor. This is

true even though few people can be unaware that drugs sometimes have unintended side effects, and a case involving babies is probably the best known example. Our knowledge of the placebo effect suggests that such trust and faith may have therapeutic benefits. Recall Anna Freud's statement that the submission, admiration, and obedience of the patient are things that "all doctors" use for the benefit of their patients. At the same time, others have expressed fears that this aspect of the doctor-patient relationship can also be used for the doctor's (but not the patient's) benefit, and, indeed, some of the findings in this study carry that implication. Patient trust in physicians in the experimental situation can have serious negative implications for informed consent, as is pointed out in Chapter Eight.

Faith in physicians, therefore, explains the ease with which some subjects decided to participate. A different aspect of the doctor-patient relationship was emphasized by one subject in explaining why she did not give the decision much consideration.

I.   Did you give serious consideration to refusing?

R.   No, I did give it some consideration, but I knew I would not refuse because I knew I was on a spot. I didn't want to get on the bad side of the doctor. (#24, white, private)

This statement once again calls attention to the dependence on the part of the patient in a relationship with a doctor, particularly in a situation in which the patient is to some degree rendered helpless by his or her condition. At such times, an expression of doubt in the physician's judgment may not be something that the patient can afford.

While factors such as a subject's relationship with her physician, usually expressed in terms of faith or confidence in him, and eagerness to have the baby were offered by subjects as explanations for their lightly-made decision regarding participation, additional data collected in the interviews allow consideration of other variables. In particular we can examine whether subjects did not take the decision seriously because they had no time to do so and because they did not fully understand the implications of the request to be in research.

As was previously mentioned, subjects learned of the research at a variety of times relative to their admission to the hospital. In the labor-induction study, the points at which subjects first learned that research was involved were distributed as follows:

3 subjects learned of research a week or more before admission
7 subjects learned 2 to 6 days before admission

8 subjects learned the day before admission
1 subject learned before admission on the day of admission
11 subjects learned after admission, before the procedure began
20 subjects learned only after the induction procedure began

Several of the subjects who learned of the research before their admission to the hospital mentioned using the time before admission to make a more careful and better informed decision. For example:

R.   How much time did you give to the decision?

I.   Well, when he asked me I said OK, but then I had two days to think about it. (#41, white, clinic)

Other subjects said that they gave immediate agreement when they were asked to participate several days ahead of time, and that they then used the interim period to get additional information or to give the decision more careful thought. Two private patients reported asking the advice of other physicians with whom they had established relationships.

Subjects who learned of the research for the first time in the labor room, however, did not have the option of mulling over the decision or of asking the advice of friends or other medical personnel. Not surprisingly, then, subjects who learned about the research before their admission to the hospital were the most likely to report making a careful decision and having some difficulty with their decision. Table 9 compares the responses of subjects who knew of research before admission with those who learned about it in the labor room.

The data indicate that those who learned of the research for the first time in the labor room were less likely to report giving serious consideration to their decisions. Both lack of time for making the decision and the pressures and distractions of the business at hand were undoubtedly involved. Most definitions of "informed consent" fail to recognize that *contextual factors of time and situation are involved whenever consent is sought.* My findings suggest that it is important to informed consent that a prospective subject be given sufficient time to consider a decision. Peer review committees are probably not sufficiently sensitive to the importance of the context in which an investigator proposes to secure the "informed consent" of his subjects.

Another possible reason for lightly-made decisions was subjects' actual knowledge of the research and its risks. However, when the amount of knowledge of subjects (still excluding those who did not know of the research before their participation began) is dichotomized and crosstabulated with whether subjects knew of the research before or after admission to the

Table 9.   Percentage of Subjects, by When Learned of Research, Who Indicated No Difficulty in Deciding to Be in the Labor-Induction Study[a]

Response	Knew Research Involved Before Admission	Learned of Research After Admission
Decision was not at all difficult	79%	82%
Did not occur to subject to say no	68%	82%
Did not seriously consider refusing	74%	91%
Made up mind immediately	58%	73%
Said yes to any of the above statements	47%	73%
(N)[b]	19	11

[a] Only subjects who were aware of the research when their involvement began are included.

[b] The point at which one subject learned of the research was not determined with certainty.

hospital, little difference emerges. Of 11 subjects with little knowledge, 6 came from the 15 subjects who knew of research before hospitalization and 5 from the 11 who learned of the research in the labor room.

Furthermore, when knowledge of the research is dichotomized and cross-tabulated with the four decision-difficulty variables, there is almost no difference. Thus, it appears that the amount of knowledge (above the minimum knowledge that research was involved) had little to do with how seriously subjects treated the participation decision.

However, it is also true that in particular cases knowledge *did* play an important role. *None* of the four subjects who had no conception of the presence or absence of risks had any difficulty with their decisions. There was also anecdotal evidence that other knowledge gaps might have played a role in the lack of serious decision. One subject told how she had agreed to be a "study patient" without knowing that an experimental drug was involved; she had initially thought that it only meant some observations and extra monitoring of her labor. She learned of the true nature of the study in the labor room, but felt the decision had already been made. Thus, the decision ease she reported referred to a decision made on partial information:

I. How difficult would you say the decision was?

R. Well, at that point it wasn't difficult, but as I said, if I had known everything ahead of time, I probably wouldn't have participated. Knowing me.

I. When you were asked to participate—did it occur to you to say no?

R. No, because I didn't know a drug was involved. I just thought it was . . . [trailed off]. (#19, white, private)

Another subject told how her physician had thought she should be induced and had suggested that she enter the hospital in the study because it was the fastest way she could be admitted. She agreed, but her response to the decision-difficulty items indicated that her ease with the decision had its basis in her lack of understanding of the research nature of her induction:

I. How much thought did you give to the decision?

R. I didn't give it very much thought. I just thought, you know, if you had to be induced, they had to take you in.

I. Would you say you made a separate decision to be in the research or was the decision to be induced and the decision to be in the research all one decision?

R. Well, the research didn't bother me in the least. I just thought that they researched on everybody if they were using the machine [she is referring either to the infusion pump or the monitoring equipment] because I was having the machine used. (#40, white, private)

This patient thought that since she was going to be in research, everyone having the procedure (labor-induction) was in research. Her decision ease was undoubtedly influenced by her belief that the researchers' request was completely routine.

In summary, the major finding discussed in this section was that most subjects had little difficulty in deciding to participate and reported making immediate decisions. The ease of their decisions, however, was perhaps not appropriate to a situation where an experimental drug was being used. Several factors seemed to be related to the lack of many seriously made decisions to participate. Educational differences in subjects and differences in the time available for the decision were related to this. Perhaps most important, however, were subjects' trust in their doctors and their eagerness to get into the hospital and have their baby.

Before leaving the topic of the ease or difficulty of decisions to be research subjects, let us briefly examine the responses of subjects in the starvation-abortion study. Most of these subjects also seemingly had little difficulty. One subject indicated decision difficulty on all four items. None of the others indicated that they had seriously considered refusing, and only one reported any difficulty at all in making the decision. Three reported they had given it "some thought," but had no other difficulty. The results of these seven subjects on the four items can be summarized as follows:

2 reported no difficulty on any item
4 reported difficulty on one item
1 reported difficulty on all four items

Thus, once again the major impression was that subjects generally did not find the decision very difficult. Risk was less of a factor in this study, but physical discomfort was a far more important consideration than in the labor-induction drug study. In explaining their responses to the four items, subjects in the starvation-abortion study offered comments similar to those of labor-induction subjects. Two explicitly mentioned the reason for their ease of decision was their eagerness to get into the hospital for their abortions.

R. The decision wasn't difficult at all. I was dying to get in. I was tired of waiting around. (#101, white)

I. Did it occur to you to say no?

R. No, it didn't because it was my first offer of getting into the hospital and getting it over with. I hadn't really thought about the three days [without eating]. Just getting in here, that's all I wanted. I just jumped at it. (#102, black)

Another starvation subject's comments indicated the potential importance of having time for a participation decision, time that was often not available to subjects in the labor-induction study:

I. How much thought did you give to the decision?

R. I thought about it because after I talked to the lady at the [abortion counseling] office, I thought about it until the doctor called up [to officially seek her agreement]. I had a whole day before the doctor called. (#104, black)

A second subject told me how she had agreed on the telephone, knowing that until she was admitted she would be able to change her mind. It was this subject who reported the most difficulty with her decision.

The concerns expressed by subjects who *did* have difficulty with their decisions were for the most part quite appropriate to each study. Reasons for hesitation mentioned by the starvation-abortion subjects concerned the physical discomfort of not eating and the extra three days of hospitalization required by participation. These costs were uppermost in subjects' minds. In the labor-induction study, neither of these factors was present. The issues here were whether induction itself was desirable and the unknown risks of an experimental drug. And it was these two issues that were consistently mentioned by the few women who reported that their decision to participate was neither simple nor easily made.

KNOWLEDGE OF STUDY

Prospective subjects' knowledge about the research in which they are asked to participate has a bearing on two topics that are examined in upcoming chapters. Such knowledge may affect subjects' reasons for participating, and it largely determines whether their participation is based upon informed consent. Accordingly, I questioned subjects about their knowledge of the study in which they were participating or had participated. Despite the claim made by some writers that "professional expertise" is necessary to judge whether or not informed consent takes place, I found that it was relatively simple to determine what most subjects did or did not understand about the research.

Since I was also interested in subjects' awareness of the extent of their own understanding of the research, I first questioned them about their *feelings of understanding*. Many labor-induction subjects knew that there were elements of the study that they did not understand.

	No Response*	Yes	No
Did you feel that you had all the information you needed or wanted in order to make your decision?	8	30	13
Were there any aspects of the study that you felt you did not understand (at the time it was started)?	7	20	24

Thus, 30 percent (13 of 43) of the labor-induction subjects responding said they did not feel they had all of the information they wanted or needed to make their decision, and 45 percent said there were aspects of the study they did not understand.

The majority did report that they felt they had enough information and that they understood the study. However, it would be a serious error to assume that they did in fact have the necessary information or that they really did understand the study. For example, of the 12 responding subjects who were *not even aware* that research was taking place until their inductions had begun, 8 reported that they had all the information they needed or wanted. Responses to the second item from this same category of unknowing subjects showed similar results—8 of 13 unknowing subjects who responded said there were *no* aspects they did not understand. In reality, of course, they understood virtually nothing about it.

It has been suggested that there may be people who "just don't want to know" and who may therefore "refuse to listen."[14] This sort of psychological defense would presumably be most likely to occur in situations where patients are particularly fearful, and in which heavy reliance on authority can be expected. Evidence presented later shows that a "refusal to listen" explanation does not account for the shortcomings in informed consent in the labor-induction study. Nevertheless, this interesting point has not been adequately addressed in the literature on human experimentation. One legal commentator has raised the issue in reference to medical malpractice, noting that "if a squeamish individual would rather not know about the potential hazards of treatment, he may delegate control to his physician through a conscious, knowing waiver."[15] (Such a waiver

---

* All of those not responding to these two items were subjects who were not aware of the research. The remainder of such subjects did respond to the two items, although it would seem that the items might not have made much sense to them under the circumstances. See Appendix B, items 72 and 73.

did not exist in the labor-induction study). The extent to which there are patients who "would rather not know" is, so far as I am aware, undocumented. The implications on disclosure of doctors' believing that patients really do not want to know are substantial. Myers, the legal commentator quoted above, recognized this and stated the implications well:

> the doctor who proceeds under the doctor-knows-best theory without securing a deliberate waiver from his patient and without disclosing collateral hazards substitutes his judgment about the desirability of undergoing risk for that of his patient. Such substitution is inconsistent with the law's respect for the patient's control over his own body . . .[16]

In a purely experimental situation, it would appear to be particularly hazardous from a legal and ethical standpoint to withhold an explanation on the grounds that the subject "might really not wish to know."

Subjects were asked one other series of questions concerning their *feelings* of understanding about various aspects of the study. These more specific questions better reflected the extent of ignorance about the study.

Table 10 shows that the amount of self-perceived knowledge about the labor-induction research varied greatly. A large proportion of the subjects felt they had no understanding of several aspects of the research. Between 40 and 50 percent of the subjects indicated *no* understanding of risks, benefits to themselves and to science, and the technical aspects of the research. The "role" item seemed not to have been understood by some subjects.

Once again the caveat must be applied that the expressed understanding of subjects on these items is not the same thing as real understanding. Subjects who had little or no understanding of the research sometimes believed that they understood things completely. Therefore, it seemed appropriate to attempt to determine exactly how much subjects actually knew about the research in which they were participating. Since these items and responses dealt with some of the details of the labor-induction research, it might be useful to briefly recapitulate the study procedures.

The double-blind study involved an experimental drug and a standard drug for inducing labor. One of these drugs was selected for each subject in a randomized process and was administered through an infusion pump that controlled the rate of flow. The experimental drug was based on a natural, hormonal substance, and, although no risks were known, it was an investigatory drug (FDA Phase 3). Each subject's labor was closely observed, and electronic fetal monitoring equipment was used in the later stages of labor. Blood samples for research purposes were taken at specified times, particu-

Table 10.   Subjects' Feelings of Understanding of Various Aspects of the Labor-Induction Study

Before the Research Started, How Well Did You Feel You Understood:[a]	No Response	Under-stood Completely	Under-stood Fairly Well	Didn't Under-stand Very Well	Didn't Under-stand at All
What was to be done	6	12	20	11	2
Any risks that might be involved	1	18	10	—	22
The potential benefits to yourself	—	14	11	3	23
The potential benefits to science—what they hoped to learn	—	8	10	7	26
Your role—what was expected of you	—	17	10	3	21
The technical aspects of the research	—	6	13	8	24

[a] All items are as read to respondents. See Appendix B, item 74.

larly following delivery and the next day. In a separate, but closely related study, a pediatrician was observing the babies delivered in the study and was running routine tests for several hours after birth. Separate consent was sought for this study, usually after a subject was well into her labor or shortly after birth. Finally, guidelines were set up governing how long an attempt to induce labor would last, that is, when the drug infusion would be stopped and the attempt considered unsuccessful. There the study ended. There were also well-understood options as to what could be done at that point. These included Caesarian section, a second attempt at induction, or dismissal from the hospital, depending upon the circumstances.

In the first few interviews, my attempt to determine how much subjects knew about the research consisted of an open-ended question that asked them to describe the study. As might have been predicted, this procedure was not satisfactory since many people's ability to describe the study did not accurately reflect the extent of their understanding. For others, it was impossible to tell from their response just what and how much they understood. The need for specific questions to determine the extent of labor-induction subjects' knowledge is well illustrated in the following typical responses to the open-ended question, "Could you tell me a little about the study—what's it all about? What do you have to do in it?"

R. I don't know. They explained it to me, but I don't know if I am using a new one or an old one or what. She said there was two kinds. An old and a new. But I don't know whether I'm getting the old one or the new one. And I don't understand what kind it is in the first place. But I just go along with what they know is best. (#20, black, clinic)

R. Not very much. It's just a drug and they give it to you. They start out slowly. And it doesn't work on some people if you are not ready. They score you and if you get such and such a score then maybe you'll have the baby, you know. But it just brings on the contractions, and then over a long period of time they keep giving you more of the drug. That's about all I know about it.

I. OK. Are they using more than one drug in the study?

R. Yes. They are using two drugs, and one, they think, works better than the other. I can't even think of what it's called. (#23, white, clinic)

R. I know very little actually. I just . . . the doctor said they were having this study where they are using three different drugs. And they might be using any one of the three. And that's about it. (#34, white, private)

R. Really, I don't know anything about it, but you don't have to do anything, you know, in it. They just put you on it. It's good. It's really good. Well . . . it's working out well so far.

I. What do you know about the drug they are using?

R. Nothing at all. I didn't read anything on it. They told me that it just starts things going, but as far as what it is . . . I haven't the slightest idea.

I. Did they tell you which drug they were using to induce labor?

R. I don't remember what she said.

I. Who?

R. The nurse that was with me. I signed the form. They explained that they are using this drug in a study.

I. Did they explain that they are comparing two different drugs?

R. Yes.

I. Did they tell you which one you are getting?

R. I don't remember if he told me which one I was getting, but I remember seeing on the paper that there were two that they used. I can't remember if they did say what they were using now . . . (#12, white, private)

I. Could you tell me what you know about it?

R. Well, from what Dr. H [house staff] said, it's been used about 5 years. And there has been about 50 women that have had this. And it seems to work better but they are trying to see how much better. And it doesn't seem to affect the baby or hurt the baby in any way. And that's as much as I really understand. (#33, white, clinic)

I. What do you know about the study?

R. I don't know anything about it. He just said that it would start labor. I don't know anything about the drug.

I. Did you sign a piece of paper about the drug?

R. Yes.

I. Did you read it pretty carefully or did you just go over it?

R. I read it, but it didn't make much sense. (#16, black, clinic)

These quotes illustrate several points. First, although these subjects were among the most articulate, it would obviously be extremely difficult to try to make any comparative judgments about their relative degree of understanding of the study on the basis of these responses to an open-ended question. The subjects quoted above actually cover the complete range in understanding of the research. One subject, the first one quoted, did not know research was involved, although she talked about the "new drug." The last subject quoted turned out to be aware she was taking part in research, though her knowledge was rather limited. And detailed questions showed that the third one quoted (who said she knew little other than that there were three drugs involved) knew quite a lot about the study. The fourth quote illustrates that specific questioning could uncover much greater understanding of the study than was in evidence solely on the subject's response to the initial question.

Second, with an open-ended question, subjects focused on a wide variety of aspects of the research, and often confined their response to the first aspect they thought of. This rendered impossible any ready comparison of relative knowledge solely on the basis of these responses.

Thus, because open-ended questions could elicit rather similar responses from subjects with large differences in understanding, and because responses tended to be focused on one or two aspects of the research rather than on the overall picture, it became evident that a series of questions dealing with specific elements of the research was necessary if any judgments or comparisons about subjects' relative understanding of the research were to be made.

Accordingly, subjects were asked, in a series of items, if they had understood 11 different aspects of the labor-induction research before the drug infusion had begun. The number of nonresponses on these items reflects the fact that these items were added after the first nine interviews had been completed. In these cases, where it could be determined elsewhere in the interview that a subject was aware of a particular element, a positive response was coded even though the specific question had not been asked. Where such a determination could not be made, it was coded as a nonresponse. This has the effect of artificially inflating the percentage (though not the number) of subjects who appeared to be aware of each element, since it meant that only a positive response could be coded for these few subjects. Nevertheless, the responses to these items, shown in Table 11, indicate that a large percentage of the subjects did not understand many of the elements of the research.

Perhaps a few words should be said about the possible role of memory failure as a factor accounting for the large numbers of subjects who indicated no knowledge of several aspects of the labor-induction research. Anyone who has taught is aware from reading students' exams that much

Table 11. Subjects' Knowledge of the Labor-Induction Study

Before the Research Started, Did You Know (or Was It Your Understanding):[a]	No Response	Yes	No	Percent of Respondents Not Knowing of Aspect Before Began
That a new drug was to be used or might be used or not	1	45	5	10%
That they were using more than one drug or not	1	39	11	22%
How the drug was to be given	8	30	13	30%
What kind of drug it was (or anything about it)	4	5	42	89%
If any risks were involved or not	2	29	20	41%
If they were going to do any special monitoring or observing of your labor or not	6	16	29	64%
If they were going to do any special observing or studying of the baby after it was born	8	8	35	81%
If they were going to do any special or extra tests (like blood tests) on you	7	8	36	82%
How long they would continue to try if it didn't work at first	9	9	33	79%
What would happen if it didn't work	9	10	32	76%

[a] Again, all items are as presented to subjects. See Appendix B, item 77.

of what is "taught" is not "learned," that is, some students will miss the point, get the information garbled, or have no recollection at all. However, I believe that memory failure is not an important factor in the present context for several reasons.

First, in this project we are not dealing with large quantities of information but rather with materials that could be covered in a 5-minute discussion. Second, the period of recall was quite short; subjects were interviewed a day or two after their labor was induced. Third, and perhaps most importantly, the form that questioning takes can influence recall. It would be one thing, for example, to ask subjects to "tell everything you knew about the research before it began" and to assume that anyone who failed to mention risks knew nothing about risks. It is quite another to ask such specific questions as "Were there any risks involved?" and "Do you recall being told anything about risks?" Under such conditions the probability seems high that a subject who gives a negative response was either not told at all, was not told in a way that he or she was capable of understanding, or was not told under circumstances that allowed for even minimally effective communication to take place. Such factors are clearly the investigator's responsibility. Thus, I do not believe that memory failure by subjects accounts for a significant amount of the lack of knowledge of the study evidenced by subjects.

Before discussing subjects' responses to these questions about the research, a word should be said about why subjects were questioned about these particular elements of the research, and a caveat must be offered about what their responses mean vis-à-vis the issue of informed consent. The questions were selected on the basis of what seemed to me to be important that subjects understood. My judgment in this regard was influenced by statements such as the FDA's, which says that researchers should "make known" to subjects:

> the nature, duration, and purpose of the administration of investigational drugs; the method and means by which it is to be administered; all inconveniences and hazards reasonably to be expected, including the fact, where applicable, that the person may be used as a control; the existence of alternative forms of therapy, if any, and the effects upon his health or person that may possibly come from the administration of the investigational drug.[17]

However, the reader should remember that the question of precisely which aspects of research must be understood by subjects before their consent can be considered to be informed is by its nature judgmental.[18] Thus, it should not be assumed that all questions asked of subjects tap an area that "current ethical standards" hold to be necessary to *informed* consent. Statements like the FDA's are subject to some interpretation in specific cases, and, furthermore, there is disagreement within the research ethics literature about which general elements of research an informed subject must understand. (The issue of blind experiments is a good example.) Since my purpose here is primarily to describe rather than prescribe, I shall not argue that subjects needed to have knowledge about all aspects in order for their consent to be considered "informed," although on some aspects, such as knowledge of risks, there might be little question.

I do believe that it would have been *desirable* for subjects to understand all of the elements about which I questioned them, but the reader can decide whether, for example, the 64 percent who did not know that special monitoring and observation would be done during their labor therefore did not give informed consent. Opinions differ on matters such as this. One of the purposes of peer review committees is, after all, to bring group judgment to bear on questions about what specific elements of a particular research project must be communicated to subjects in order to satisfy the general requirements of the FDA statement.*

Subjects' knowledge and a discussion of that knowledge are presented later in this chapter. The implications of this knowledge on participation decisions and on the reasons why subjects participate and on the issue of informed consent are dealt with in later chapters. Let us turn to subjects' knowledge of the items in Table 11.

New Drug. The first item in Table 11, "Did you know if a new drug was to be used or might be used?" needs clarification. Forty-five of 50 responding subjects said they knew a "new drug" was involved. However, since 20 women did not know that research was involved until after their inductions had begun, many of these 45 women obviously did not understand that this "new drug" was experimental. "New drug" simply did not mean "experimental drug" to many subjects. This euphemism, however, was constantly used by all persons connected with the research, and found its way into my questionnaire.

"New drug," of course, is a positively valued term. Many subjects assumed it meant "proven." Television and other advertising has probably irrevocably linked the terms "new" and "better" in many minds. "Experimental," however, is something else, and conjures up images of mad scientists on the late show and the dangers of the unknown. For this reason, it is perhaps understandable that the term "experimental" was avoided. That this avoidance was intentional became evident when I was explicitly warned against using the term by one of the research nurses. She said that it might alarm subjects, even though the subjects I interviewed had supposedly already given their informed consent—that is, they had all signed consent forms—before I interviewed them.

While it might seem obvious that the term "new drug" would seem innocent or even favorable to many patients, it was a research subject who

---

* In the case of the labor-induction study, the review committee's judgment is reflected in the consent form, which is reprinted in Appendix A.

first brought this to my attention:*

I. When did you first realize it was research? When I first came to talk to you about it or before?

R. Right. When you came in to talk to me. That was when I really found out the whole story of what it was all about, you know.

I. Up until that time?

R. I knew that they was going to use a new drug, but I didn't know they was testing this drug out, you know. (#20, black, clinic)

Thus, five subjects did not know that a new drug might be used. Fifteen knew that a *new* drug was involved but did not understand that it was an *experimental* drug. Such an understanding appears to be basic to informed consent in this (or any other) drug study.

Incidentally, little is known about what the words "experimental drug" connote for patients. The research staff's avoidance of the term suggests that they believed the word "experimental" might evoke unrealistic images or irrational fears. I have seen little evidence, either in my own study or in the literature, that such reactions are a significant problem. However, if ordinary people do harbor unrealistically negative conceptions of "experiments," researchers must face this problem, rather than evading it by misleading subjects. There are good reasons to believe that requirements for informed consent will become more exacting in future years. Terms (like "new drug") that fail to communicate essential information to subjects are not consistent with the goal of informed consent. If unrealistic fears are a significant problem, the experimental situation provides investigators with excellent opportunities to educate the lay public. Most people, for example, are probably not aware of the stages through which an investigational drug must pass before it is used on human subjects.

Which Drug Would Be Used.   While 78 percent of the labor-induction sub-

* It was not until almost 30 interviews had been completed that I became aware that I had perhaps assumed erroneously that some subjects knew of the research because they had indicated their awareness that "new drugs" were involved. It was necessary to telephone several subjects who had already been interviewed to determine whether any misunderstandings had occurred because of this ambiguity. The responses of two subjects had to be reinterpreted when I discovered that they had not known of the research before my first interview with them, but had learned of it inadvertently from something I had said during that interview. At that time my impression had been that they knew about the research because they had told of reading the consent form or because they had known that a "new drug" was involved.

jects knew that more than one drug was involved in the study, most did not understand how the assigning of a drug to a subject was determined. Sixty-nine percent of the subjects did not understand that a double-blind methodology was being used.* This information was elicited by asking subjects who knew that more than one drug was being used in the study if they knew which drug was used in their case. A lack of understanding on this point was usually quite obvious:

I. Did you know what drug they would actually use?

R. No.

I. Did you know that it was part of the research that you didn't know?

R. I thought they forgot to tell me. (#38, white, clinic)

Although not even the investigators or nurses knew which drug each subject was receiving, at least nine subjects assumed that they were receiving a particular drug—the new one. Perhaps some could not divorce the idea of being in research from the idea of getting the new drug. In any event, as they talked about this, the positive valuation of the term "new drug" was apparent:

R. They are *letting me* try the new one. (my emphasis) (#17, black, clinic)

R. . . . they have been using one particular drug in past years for inducement, and they have come up with new ones. And because I had been induced before—it was my fourth—they were going to try one of the two† newer ones, but he didn't know just what particular one it would be. (#29, white, private)

Others incorrectly assumed the choice of the drug they received would depend on their own needs. Hence:

* This information is not shown in Table 11, although it came from the series of questions shown in that table (see item 77 in Appendix B). Subjects' awareness of the double-blind aspect was determined through follow up questions to the item "Did you know what drug they would actually use?" Since the correct answer was "no," and the interpretation of that answer required probing, it made little sense to include the item in Table 11.

† The subject's reference to two new drugs resulted from the fact that the consent form was not updated after one of the two experimental drugs was withdrawn from the study before the interviews for the present study began. At the time the interviews were done, two drugs—an experimental and the standard one—were being used in the study.

R. I interpreted it as there were three different kinds of drugs to be given, and they would use the one they thought would be best in your, you know, your condition or whatever. (#36, white, private)

R. I assumed it—the drug selected—would be the best for me. (#38, white, private)

I. How did you think they were going to decide which drug to give you? Did you know?

R. Well, I figured they would take into consideration, you know, my condition and what was happening with me.

I. That's what I was wondering, because several people told me they figured they would get the drug best for them.

R. Yeah. I certainly thought *I* was taken into consideration. (#44, black, clinic)

One subject who discovered shortly before her induction began that she might not receive the new drug was particularly disturbed about it. She had come to understand from her doctor that he was allowing her to be induced only because the new drug would speed her labor and lessen the risk to which the standard drug would subject her. During the first interview it was apparent that both she and her husband were upset, but the reason for their agitation was expressed more clearly during the second interview, after the successful delivery of their baby:

R. Dr. D [private physician] wanted to check me Monday afternoon before he recommended it [induction]. And after he checked me he didn't think that I should do it because he thought I would go another week and that I'd be in labor too long. He didn't think I was ready. But then Tuesday, he called and said that they had a new drug. *That's* what the thing is. He didn't recommend that I come in with the old drug, but since they had a *new* drug that would probably work better.*

---

* The source of this subject's misunderstanding on this point is not clear, because I do not know what her physician actually told her. It is not likely that her physician had an erroneous understanding of the research, because the principal investigator reported having explained the research in detail to house staff and private physicians at the time he solicited their cooperation in locating subjects. Furthermore, this particular private physician had close professional ties with the principal investigator, as was described earlier.

And then when I came in I found out that I might not even have that drug—see? That I might go through a day of agony and not deliver. But, I think that they were just lucky that I'm one that delivers fast or it might not have worked. (#04, white, private)

Interestingly, not all subjects who were aware of the blind methodology had been *told* about it, as the following highly sophisticated subject indicated:

I. Did you know what drug they would actually use?

R. I thought that they might not even know themselves. See, I didn't know how they were doing this. I thought maybe everything was sort of coded and only afterwards . . .

I. Did they tell you that?

R. No. No. No. I was just thinking that sometimes in these things they don't want to know beforehand; they just want to see the results. And then, after the whole thing is done . . .

I. That's what they did.

R. I guess I'm a little bit acquainted with this kind of thing. (#34, white, private)

The researchers apparently made no special effort to tell most subjects about the double-blind aspect of the study, though it does not seem to have been concealed. How so many subjects could not know about it can be better understood from the following account of how one subject learned of the double-blind aspect:

I. Did you know about the two drugs before they started the infusion?

R. I found out when they were getting it hooked up. I said, "Now what is the name of this drug?" and he said "It is either this or this." I asked, "You don't know which one it is?" and he told me that it was a double-blind study. So he was putting it in the machine but he hadn't actually hooked it up yet. But I had already signed the paper. (#04, white, private)

The double-blind aspect of the research, then, appears to have been learned almost incidently or, in some cases, guessed at by well-educated subjects familiar with research techniques. This being the case, it is understandable that relatively few subjects knew about it.

With regard to the "kind of drug" that was being tested, only a handful (5 of 42 responding) knew anything about the type of substance it was. These subjects learned as a result of their own curiosity and from asking direct questions about it. Most subjects, when asked about the "kind of drug" that was being used, responded by telling me the purpose of the drug:

R. I didn't know anything more than the fact that it was an inducing agent. (#32, white, private)

Understanding of Risks. The researchers described the project in the consent form as having no *known* risks; as an experimental drug, it could not properly be described otherwise.

Interpretation of subjects' responses to the questions concerning risk was difficult, because there seemed to be little correspondence between a subject's indicating that she had been specifically informed about the question of risks and her response as to whether there were risks involved or not. In other words, some subjects who indicated that there were "no *known* risks" seemed to have figured it out themselves, while some who said there were "no risks" had been given some information about this. Furthermore, the distinction between "no risks" and " no known risks" may not have been meaningful for many subjects. Therefore, only subjects who said they did not know *anything* about risks are included in the 41 percent having no knowledge of risks in Table 11. A few responses from such subjects follow:

I. How much thought did you give to risks?

R. No. I didn't think about it. I wasn't worried; I know they have good doctors here.

I. Did they say anything about risks, one way or the other?

R. No. Nobody told me there was any risks or that there wasn't any risks. (#07, white, clinic)

I. How well did you feel you understood any risk that might have been involved?

R. I didn't know really. It never crossed my mind. (#21, black, clinic)

I. Were any risks involved, or not?

R. No. They didn't tell me about any risks. Were there any risks? (#47, black, clinic)

Turning to subjects who did have some knowledge about risks, we again find striking expressions of faith and trust in physicians, to the point where assumptions of no risk were made when apparently no knowledge was present:

I. How well did you feel you understood any risks that might be involved?

R. I guess I assumed, you know, that everything they'd be using was already safe, and that they just wanted to see different reactions. But that they weren't, you know, going to try anything that might really not be safe. I must say that I probably thought about it a little more afterwards than I did at the time. Somehow I didn't connect it with all the things I usually do about new drugs, because I am very skeptical about this kind of thing. I always feel that . . . well, at that time they think it's so and then later on things happen. But I just really didn't think about it at all. (#34, white, private)

R. I assumed that there were no risks. My assumption. Nobody actually came out and said there were no risks. That inherited childhood faith in medicine, right? I should know better, but I just rallied forth this time. (#49, white, private)

R. I just assumed there weren't any [risks]. Again, because of [faith in] my own doctor. (#32, white, private)

R. In respect to safety and everything, I would imagine that they wouldn't try it at all if they didn't feel that it was as safe as it could possibly be.

I. Are you assuming that, or did they say so?

R. I'm assuming that this would probably be it. Since they are people in the medical profession and are interested in saving life, not taking it away, I would imagine that they wouldn't do anything or use any drugs that would be known to have ill effects . . . I had no question as to whether it would be as safe as it could possibly be. (#30, white, clinic)

Many subjects who believed there were no risks did say that this is what they had been told (although it must be remembered that I have no data on what was actually said). These repeated comments reflect a fundamental lack of understanding of the nature of research using experimental drugs:

R.   He said it wasn't harmful and wouldn't cause any damage. (#09, black, clinic)

R.   He told me there was no risks involved. I put my confidence in him. (#11, white, clinic)

R.   Dr. V [house staff] told me that I didn't have anything to worry about. (#14, white, clinic)

R.   The doctor told me there was no harm, so I guess there was no risk. (#20, black, clinic)

R.   Dr. V [house staff] said there wouldn't be any harm. (#23, white, clinic)

R.   Oh, they said there wasn't any risk, so I took their word for it. (#16, white, clinic)

R.   The only thing I ever worried about—the first thing that popped into my mind—was would it harm the baby. That was quickly relieved. (#03, white, private)

All eight of these women indicated that they had been *told*, not that they had assumed, that there were no risks. It is possible, however, that a statement about "no known risks" became "no risks" in their minds.

Only two subjects said they had been informed that there was some chance of risk.

I. Were there any risks of complications involved?

R. No. [pause] Well, there were risks. They said there were risks. Right? You never know. Like they say, there are always risks with a new drug.

I. Not everyone realizes that.

R. Actually there is a risk in almost any kind of drug you take. (#12, white, private)

R. They said there were very few risks involved. That 9 times out of 10 there wouldn't be any. And that's usually the way it is anyway. [laughed] (#30, white, clinic).

The "9 times out of 10" may have referred to the probability that the induction would result in the delivery of the baby, not the probability of harm, which was the focus of my question. The tendency of subjects to confuse the research and nonresearch aspects of their induction will be examined later.

Finally, two subjects who recognized the possibility of risks indicated that they assumed the possibility rather than having been informed about it:

R. Sure, I could have reacted to the drug as with any drug. (#02, white, clinic)

R. There is always the chance I'd be the first one. (#24, white, private)

In summary, several things can be said about the labor-induction subjects' knowledge of risks. First, many (41 percent) knew nothing about risks and made no assumptions about them. Second, many more believed no risks were present. Some seemed to have assumed this, but the majority said that this was what they had been told. Third, relatively few recognized the possibility of unknown risk, and only two indicated that they had been informed on this possibility. An understanding of risks would seem to be a fundamental aspect of informed consent in this study. In these terms, such consent was a rare commodity.

The discussion thus far has proceeded as if knowledge of risks can easily be imparted from researcher to subject. The communications problems have not been studied very much, but the matter is probably more complicated than implied by this discussion. A sophisticated conception of risks must recognize that risk is relative and must be measured against some standard to have meaning. The few subjects who noted that all drugs carry risks at some level of probability were of course correct. (In addition, what will be perceived as risky is to some extent situationally specific. Procedures that would be risky for a healthy individual might not seem risky to the individual for whom the procedure is a final hope.) Despite the relative nature of medical risks, I suspect that comparatively few laymen ordinarily think of medical risk in relative terms; something either is or is not "risky." If this is true, then researchers' statements that there are minimal risks or no known risks may be translated by subjects as "no risks." This would be particularly likely if the risk is attached to a course of action to which one is already committed. In the absence of a careful study of subjects' understanding of risks in situations in which special attention has been paid to communicating a realistic understanding of risk, it is difficult to know how important this factor may be.[19]

The possibility that some laymen think of risk in relativistic terms raises the interesting question of the standard against which risk is ordinarily judged. If experience provides the standard, then the answer probably lies in what doctors ordinarily communicate to patients about risks. So far as I know, there have been no studies of physician disclosure of risks in such ordinary situations as the drug prescribing of everyday medical practice.

One other issue must be acknowledged in this discussion of subjects' understanding of risks. Most ethical statements and policy guidelines stress the investigator's responsibility with regard to disclosing risks to prospective subjects. While communication between researcher and subject may be difficult with regard to such matters as risk, it must also be recognized that keeping subjects' understanding of risks at a minimum may be useful to investigators in their efforts to recruit and retain subjects. Because subjects' ignorance can make it easier for the researcher to do his work, it may be unrealistic to expect researchers to make more than perfunctory efforts to "inform" subjects about matters that might make subjects hesitate to participate. As things now stand, researchers are expected voluntarily to take actions that may not seem to be in their short-run interests, because subjects might be harder to recruit. We should probably not be surprised when happily participating research subjects turn out to not understand the risks of the procedure to which they are being exposed. The social control implications of situations in which people are expected to voluntarily (without supervision) take actions that make their work more difficult will be examined in more detail in the final chapter.

Special Monitoring and Extra Blood Samples.   In addition to the use of an experimental drug, the special monitoring (including fetal monitoring) and the blood samples required from subjects were elements of the research that directly affected subjects. However, Table 11 shows that most subjects did not know about these two items. Sixty-four percent of the labor-induction subjects did not know of special monitoring, and 82 percent did not know that several blood samples were to be taken in the research at the time their participation began. Again, the implications for informed consent seem clear.

Observation of the Baby.   Since the pediatrician's study of the baby for a 6-hour period after delivery was a separate study, with separate consent requested, I did not give that aspect of the study close attention. In fact, I was well into the interviewing period before I learned it was being done. However, it became apparent that the consent procedures being used in that study also had difficulties.

Although I did not seek much information from subjects about this study, it became clear in the interviews that, in most cases, subjects were not being told before their induction began that a study involving their babies was contemplated. In fact, an early subject asked me about it:

R.   Could I ask you a question before we go on? How come they put the baby under observation for 6 hours? It was because of the research, wasn't it? (#08, white, clinic)

As is shown in Table 11, only 8 of 43 labor-induction subjects knew of this aspect of the research before their inductions began. It was not clear to me whether a specific procedure was being followed concerning the point in the induction process at which the question of a baby's participation in the further study was raised, but a number of women reported learning of this at about the time their baby was born. "I was told that just before I delivered" (#19, black, clinic). Similar statements from several other subjects lead me to believe that this was a common pattern. This procedure had a startling effect on one subject.

I.   Did you know before they started if they were going to do any special monitoring or studying of the baby after it was born?

R. I didn't know about that until just before I went in to have the baby. Immediately before. And I'm afraid that's the only part that disturbed me a little bit. Because the doctors came in and all of a sudden said, "We are taking the baby for 6 hours observation afterward." And that bothered me. That's the only part of the whole thing that bothered me. And I actually completely *stopped* my labor for about 15 minutes.

I. Really?

R. Absolutely no labor. It was right in the middle of a contraction when he said it, and it just stopped. Nothing. The doctor said it was a perfect example of adrenalin being produced, that it would stop labor. Because he said they've said this through research that an abnormal flow of adrenalin in a person will stop labor. And that's exactly what happened. It stopped. No contractions for 15 minutes.

I. What happened then?

R. Well, after I had calmed down they told me that I didn't have to agree to their taking the baby, that I could have the baby with me. Then after they had explained that to me and fixed that for me, then I relaxed a little more and the contractions started back up again. It was really amazing. My heartbeat slowed down and everything.

I. So then you kept the baby with you afterwards?

R. Yes. But you see, it would have been a different story if he had just said "if there are any complications with the baby or anything—we just want to monitor the baby to make sure. This is just a test procedure with us, it will help us in our research." But he didn't say that. It sounded like all of a sudden they were expecting something to happen. And that kind of scared me.

I. Perhaps it was just the lack of advance warning?

R. Right.

I. They must have overlooked it when they were telling you the rest.

R. Well, as a matter of fact, the nurse said that they don't usually mention it to patients until afterwards. So I didn't particularly appreciate it at all. (#30, white, clinic)

A second difficulty with the consent-seeking procedure in the baby study was that—like the labor-induction study itself—some subjects did not recognize the request for cooperation in a research project for what it was. A possible explanation is that it may not have been phrased as a request.

I. Did you know before they started if they were going to do any special monitoring or studying of the baby after it was born?

R. Yes.

I. Did you know that before they started?

R. I'm trying to think at what point Dr. J [the pediatrician doing the study] came in. He came in about while I was being induced. I can't remember whether this was when they were giving me the anesthetic or not. But he told me who he was and that they were going to observe the baby. But I don't know at that point if it really dawned on me why. I mean, it didn't alarm me. I just thought it might be because I was being induced—that it was just something that they did. And I was very pleased. (#36, white, private)

There was a greater likelihood that women would refuse to cooperate in the pediatrics study than in their own labor-induction study. Some of the reasons for this emerge in the following interview excerpt:

I. Did you know before they started if they were going to do any special monitoring or studying of the baby after it was born?

R. No.

I. Did they, do you know?

R. Not that I know of.

I. Was the baby with you right afterwards, or not?

R. Yeah. They just cleaned her—gave her a bath and everything—and then they gave her to me.

I. I asked because they were observing some babies for 6 hours after birth.

R.   They asked me if I wanted this done, but I didn't. I said no. In fact, I didn't even ask my husband. But it would have been a matter of we couldn't have seen her; they would take her immediately. And [laughing] after I had a girl I was not about to have her . . .

I.   Did they ask you at that point?

R.   Uh . . . right before. But I wanted to see her and hold her and everything. And there was another thing about X rays or something which I didn't care for too much at such a young age. But I think it was mainly the separation thing, where we really wanted to enjoy her. (#45, white, private)

The closely-related pediatric study of the baby, then, was usually not brought to the attention of the prospective mothers until after their participation in the main study had begun. The reason for this apparently had more to do with factors of ease and convenience for the investigator than with a desire to present the study so it could be well understood by the mothers-to-be. It will later be argued that this pattern was also true of the labor-induction study itself, with the same unfortunate consequences for the goal of informed consent.

Other Knowledge of the Research.   Before leaving the topic of the labor-induction subjects' knowledge of the study, two other questions should be examined.

First, were subjects knowledgeable about the *purpose* of the research in which they were participating? In general, they were not. It was indicated earlier that more than half of the labor-induction subjects reported that they felt they "didn't understand at all" the potential benefits of the research for science. Several of their comments suggest that either they were not told about this or they did not have any time to consider this aspect.

I.   How well did you feel you understood the potential benefit to science—what they hoped to learn?

R.   I never thought about it. (#01, black, clinic)

R.   I wasn't really concerned about science at that particular point. I'm not really a great humanitarian at 7 o'clock in the morning. [laughed] (#34, white, private)

R.   I wouldn't say I understood it completely. As I said, I'm more interested in it now. It would occur to me more to think about that now. At the time, I think I was thinking purely in terms of myself. (#32, white, private)

R.   I still don't know what all this is supposed to be for. (#07, white, clinic)

This aspect of the research was also touched upon in the first interview when subjects were asked, "Why are they doing the study? What do they hope to learn?" Only 19 of 48 responding (40 percent) could give a correct answer to the question; many of these indicated that their answer was a guess.

I.   Why are they doing the study?

R.   I imagine to see if it will lessen the time of labor. (#24, white, private)

R.   I guess to see if the drug is better than the one they have been using in the past. (#11, white, clinic)

R.   To see something like, I guess, which would be an effective drug for inducing labor. (#34, white, private)

R.   Oh, I didn't go into that. I assume they want to see if they can induce people. (#32, white, private)

R.   Gee, I don't know. They didn't explain that to me. It's like I said, the only thing . . . they find out which drug works the best, the quickest. The old one or the new one. (#28, black, clinic)

Twenty-eight of the remaining responding subjects simply could not answer the question about the purpose of the study. Of course, at the time of this interview, 20 of them did not even know that a research study was underway.

Second, were subjects aware of alternatives to participation? An understanding of the choice before one is certainly an implication of the concept of informed consent, but almost half the subjects in the labor-induction study did not know what were their alternatives to participation. When asked what would have been done if they had not wanted to have their labor induced in the study, 5 subjects said they would have been induced the regular way, 19 said they would not have been induced but would have waited for their labor to begin, and 3 said they would have been induced at a later time. Many of these answers were nothing more than guesses. Twenty-four subjects said they did not know what they would have done if they had not wanted to be in the study. More details and a number of subject quotations on this important point are presented in Chapter Eight when the barriers to informed consent are examined in close detail. It will be argued that the widespread lack of knowledge of an alternative was an important shortcoming of the consent procedure in this study.

CONCLUSION

In this chapter two important topics relating to subjects' decision-making have been discussed. First, it was shown that labor-induction subjects generally gave little thought and consideration to what would seem to be an important decision involving the use of an experimental drug. Among the factors accounting for this were subjects' faith in physicians and eagerness to have their baby at the earliest possible time, educational differences among subjects, and the amount of time subjects had in which to make their decisions.

Second, we examined the knowledge upon which subjects based their decisions to participate. The erroneous assumption that decisions were actually being made by subjects was pointed out; many subjects (including the 20 who were unaware of the research when their inductions began) really made no decision to be a research subject. In addition to the subjects who were unaware of the research, it was shown that most subjects did not understand other key elements of the research, such as its double-blind nature, the presence of unknown risks with an experimental drug, the monitoring procedures and blood samples, the related study of their newborn infant, the purpose of the study, and their alternatives to participation. These all have serious implications for the authenticity of informed consent, which is addressed in Chapter Eight.

It may be worth noting that, as a nonexpert outsider, I found it relatively simple to ascertain what subjects knew about the research. Researchers should be able to do so before subjects begin to participate in their research, thereby assuring that no uninformed subjects participate. Furthermore, it would not be difficult for review committees interested in more than *prior* review to interview samples of subjects in order to make sure that investigators are properly discharging their ethical responsibilities.

NOTES

1. Paul Ramsey, *The Patient as Person—Explorations in Medical Ethics* (New Haven: Yale University Press, 1970), p. 5.

2. Jay Katz, in *Proceedings of the Conference on the Ethical Aspects of Experimentation on Human Subjects* (November 3 and 4, 1967), (Boston: American Academy of Arts and Sciences, 1968), p. 25.

3. Justice Schroeder, *Natanson* v *Kline,* 186 Kan. 393, 350 P.2d 1093 (1960). Key sections of this decision are reprinted in Jay Katz, *Experimentation with Human Beings* (New York: Russell Sage, 1973), pp. 529–535. (Quote is from p. 533.) A highly useful selection of materials on informed consent has been assembled by Katz in Chapters 8, 9, and 10 of that book. Many of the references in this chapter are to materials appearing in that most valuable book.

4. *Schloendorff* v *New York Hospital,* 211 N.Y. 127, 129, 105 N.E. 92, 93 (1914). Quote appears in Katz, *Experimentation . . . ,* p. 526.

5. Katz, *Experimentation . . . ,* p. 523.

6. L. J. Henderson, "Physician and Patient as a Social System," *New England Journal of Medicine,* 212 (1935), 819. Quote appears in Katz, *Experimentation . . . ,* p. 677.

7. W. R. Houston, "The Doctor Himself a Therapeutic Agent," *Annals of Internal Medicine,* 11 (1938), 1415. Quote appears in Katz, *Experimentation . . . ,* p. 684.

8. See, for example, Jerome D. Frank, *Persuasion and Healing* (New York: Schocken, 1963). Originally published by Johns Hopkins University Press in 1961.

9. David Mechanic, *Medical Sociology: A Selective View* (New York: Free Press, 1968), p. 189.

10. "The Doctor-Patient Relationship," in Katz, *Experimentation . . . ,* p. 635.

11. Ibid.

12. See, for example, Katz, *Experimentation . . . ,* p. 573, which reprints relevant sections of the FDA's statement of policy on "Consent for Use of Investigational New Drugs (IND) on Humans."

13. Alexander M. Capron, "The Law of Genetic Therapy," in *The New Genetics and the Future of Man,* M. Hamilton, ed. (Grand Rapids, Mich.: Eerdmans, 1972). Quotation appears in Katz, *Experimentation . . . ,* p. 575.

14. David Mechanic, personal communication, 1973.

15. Michael Justin Myers, "Informed Consent in Medical Malpractice," *California Law Review,* 55 (1967), 1407–1410. Quotation appears in Katz, *Experimentation . . . ,* p. 583.

16. Ibid.

17. Quoted in William J. Curran, "Governmental Regulation of the Use of Human Subjects in Medical Research: The Approach of Two Federal Agencies," *Daedalus,* 98 (Spring 1969), 563.

18. For example, Glass argues that in a lawsuit the question of what information should have been disclosed by a doctor is a judgment that should be made by a jury. Eleanor S.

Glass, "Restructuring Informed Consent—Legal Therapy for the Doctor-Patient Relationships," *Yale Law Journal,* 79 (1970), 1559–1562. Quotation appears in Katz, *Experimentation . . . .* p. 587.

19. An article by Epstein and Lasagna shows the potential difficulties of such an approach. They report a study in which subjects were asked to take a drug (aspirin with a disguised name). The description of the risks of the drug was varied on three different consent forms. As more details were presented to subjects—the added details consisted mainly of increasingly remote possible side effects—they were found to be increasingly unlikely to agree to take the drug. Whatever the intention of the study—other writers have cited it to show how foolish and irrational subjects are—it clearly shows the importance of a genuine effort to communicate with subjects and the difficult questions of judgment that arise regarding what must be disclosed. It also illustrates well the extent to which the subject is in a position to be manipulated at will by the investigator. Lynn Chaiklin Epstein and Louis Lasagna, "Obtaining Informed Consent: Form or Substance," *Archives of Internal Medicine,* 123 (1969), 682–688.

CHAPTER SIX

TYPES OF SUBJECTS

Two contrasting images of medical research subjects emerge from the literature. Research subjects are viewed either as colleagues or as victims of investigators. From the sparse empirical research on the topic, the clearest picture of subjects is found in Renée Fox's study of a metabolic research ward, *Experiment Perilous*.[1] The subject emerges as a somewhat heroic individual, highly committed to medical research and very interested in the research in which he is participating—research which is, in Fox's study, of life and death importance to him. Furthermore, he has an almost collegial relationship with the researchers and has tried to learn all he can about his disease and the research. He is pleased to make his contribution and to help future patients. Fox does not see such a researcher-subject relationship as exceptional. In another context, she suggests that researchers' willingness to establish a quasi-collegial relationship with subjects is one factor that makes American society conducive to medical research.[2] Some recent evidence, however, suggests that such a relationship between subject and researcher may be relatively uncommon.[3]

The other picture of research subjects emerges from the writings of critics who believe that many research subjects are not informed. To date, the most adequate documentation for this suspicion has been the published reports of studies in which there is little benefit and substantial risk to subjects. The assumption is that "except in rare cases, the reality is that patients will not knowingly put their health or their lives in jeopardy for a scientific experiment."[4] Beecher and Pappworth have both published summaries of many such published research reports, from which they infer that subjects would not have consented if they truly understood the risks involved. While their work has increased awareness of ethical problems in human experimentation, the fact that they make inferences from published reports provides no *direct* evidence that subjects are not informed. Further-more, such an approach does not furnish us with any information about the process that resulted in the consent inadequacies that were presumed to exist. We explore this in detail in Chapter Eight.

Thus, the literature suggests two types of research subjects. At one end of the continuum is the subject as colleague, committed to the research. At the other end is the subject as laboratory animal, being subjected to risks he does not understand. But does this exhaust the types of research sub-jects? Are these two types really the ends of a single continuum? What are the social antecedents of a subject's becoming any particular type of sub-ject?

My findings suggest that there are at least five different types of research subjects. Based on their stated reasons for participating and the knowledge they possess about the research, the five types are (1) *unaware subjects* who do not know they are taking part in research, (2) *unwilling subjects* who feel coerced and who would prefer not to take part, (3) *indifferent subjects* who give no reason for participating, (4) *benefiting subjects* who agree be-cause of advantages they perceive, and (5) *committed subjects* who give al-truistic reasons for agreeing to be research subjects. Much of this chapter consists of detailed descriptions of subjects in each of the categories. Unless specified otherwise, the discussion and the analysis pertain to labor-induc-tion subjects. Table 12 shows that most labor-induction subjects fell into two categories, unaware subjects and benefiting subjects, with a few in each of the other three types. All starvation-abortion subjects were either benefiting or committed subjects.

Table 12. Distribution of Subject Types in Two Medical Research Projects

Type	Labor-Induction Subjects		Starvation-Abortion Subjects	
	Number	Percent	Number	Percent
Unaware subjects	20	39	0	—
Unwilling subjects	4	8	0	—
Indifferent subjects	3	6	0	—
Benefiting subjects	22	43	5	71
Committed subjects	2	4	2	29
Total	51	100%	7	100%

UNAWARE SUBJECTS

I. Did you realize at the time they gave you the form to sign about the new drug that it was research or did it really register that it was research?

R. No. It didn't really register that it was research. Until you came in and started talking. (#10, black, clinic)

I. Did you know from the beginning that there was going to be research, or just that you would be induced?

R. I didn't know. I didn't know. 'Cause you see, the first time they mentioned it to me was last Tuesday.

I. Did he tell you then there was going to be research? Or did he just say that they would induce you?

R. That they would induce me. He didn't tell me about the research.

I. When did you first find out about the research?

R. Yesterday morning when you came.

I. When I came?

R. Yes. See, I didn't know, you know. (#18, black, clinic)

I. How did you find out about the study—meaning the research aspect of your induction? Was that this morning, or . . .

R. It was just when you said something to me about it. Otherwise I would never even . . . I wouldn't have had any idea. (#36, white, private)

These excerpts introduce a major and unanticipated finding of this study. Twenty labor-induction subjects, 39 percent of those interviewed, were not aware that research was involved in their inductions until after the drug infusion had begun, although all had signed consent forms. With the exception of one or two subjects who never did understand about the research (even after I questioned them), all of them learned of the research from me during one of my two interviews with them. It should be recalled that subjects were interviewed only *after* their participation had actually begun.

None of the starvation-abortion subjects could be considered unaware subjects. However, one woman came to the hospital not understanding that the fast was for research purposes. She learned that research was to be involved when she was admitted to a special research floor. Since she knew of the research before she actually began her fast, she was not classified as unaware.

In some cases it quickly became apparent that a subject was unaware of participating in research.

I. Did they have you sign a form by any chance that talked about drugs?

R. No. [pause] I just signed the form this morning to start labor.

I. Just to start labor? Did you read that form?

R. No, I didn't read it. She said that was what it's for, and I signed it. [laughed]

I. Did you know they'd be using a new drug?

R. Well, they used a drug. But it sure didn't help any, that's for sure.*

I. Do you remember if you signed a form that told about the drugs they would be using?

R. No. I signed a form for them to start labor was all. (#37, white, clinic)

I. I understand the way they are inducing you is that they are using a new drug. Do you know anything about that? Did they say anything?

R. No. I don't know anything about it.

I. Did they have you sign a piece of paper?

R. Yes.

I. Did you read it?

---

* This subject was one of seven for whom the labor-induction attempt was not successful.

R. Yes.

I. Did it say anything about them comparing different drugs, do you remember?

R. I can't even remember. I think this is a new one because it's not like I
had before.

I. But you don't know anything about their using a new drug other than
it is being given to you in a different way?

R. No.

I. I think we will stop here and I'll talk to you later.

. . .

I. I remember Tuesday when I talked to you I mentioned something
about a new drug and you didn't know about it . . . what I was
wondering was did you know you were part of research while you were
being induced?

R. No. (#26, black, clinic)

I. Some of the ladies I have talked to are taking part in a study where
they are comparing a new drug for inducing labor with an old drug.
Are you taking part? Did they say anything to you about that?

R. They are just inducing my labor as far as I know. I think. (#51, black,
clinic)

Thus, in some interviews it was quite obvious that subjects were participating in the research project without their knowledge. In other interviews,
however, it was sometimes difficult to determine just how much a subject
knew about the research, because of several problems—both methodological and ethical. Dealing with the ethical problem exacerbated one of the
methodological problems.

The first methodological problem resulted from a preconception on my
part. It had not occurred to me that I might encounter subjects who were
not even aware that they were taking part in research, because all of the required procedures had been followed. The approval of the Clinical Re-

search Committee had been received after the original consent form had been simplified so as to be readily understandable to the "average layman" (to the extent that committee members—most of whom had more than 6 years of specialized training beyond college—could gauge the layman's capacity for understanding). The consent form (see Appendix A) seemed to be straightforward, and was being signed by all subjects. Therefore, I was not anticipating unaware subjects, and when I first encountered one—the fifth subject I interviewed—I did not realize that she was not aware of the research. With some embarrassment, I offer the following excerpt from that interview:

I. Could you tell me a little about the study—what's it all about?

R. I don't know nothing about it.

I. What have they told you about it?

R. He just told me that it would induce labor. And that's all.

I. Did they tell you that they are using a new drug?

R. Well, they made me read a paper telling that there is two kinds of drugs. That's all I know.

I. Why did you decide to participate?

R. I don't know really.

I. Did you think about whether you wanted to be in something using a new drug or whether you wanted to do it in some other way?

R. No. The doctor just told me that I would have to come in to induce the labor. So I came in.

I. Which doctor?

R. I don't remember his name.

I. At the clinic?

R. Yes.

. . .

I. What was the project about? What did you have to do?

R. Well, I really don't know what they were doing. I mean they were trying to find out something about the blood or something. I really don't know.

   . . .

I. And when you came in, the doctor told you that they had a new drug they wanted you to use?

R. I just had to sign my name on a piece of paper saying it was OK.

I. Do you remember what was on the paper that you signed?

R. Well, it told about the two different kinds of medicines to bring on the labor and everything, but I really don't remember.

I. But you knew there were two different drugs?

R. Yes, and they would try one or the other. (#05, white, clinic)

Nowhere in my interview with this subject did I ask her if she knew that she was in a research project, or when she had learned of the research. My expectations plus the fact that she had obviously read the form and seemed to know about the "new drug" blinded me to her lack of awareness of the study. After I had done several additional interviews and had learned more about what was taking place, I telephoned her to ask whether she knew of the research, and, if so, when she had learned about it. I found out that she had learned from me, during our original interview.

However, with some unaware subjects it was impossible to overlook their lack of awareness, as some of the earlier excerpts showed. So I did not remain naive concerning the possibility of unaware subjects very long. In fact, the very next subject I interviewed was one who obviously did not know about the research:

I. Are they using a new drug with you? Did they tell you anything like that or do you remember?

R. No.

I. They are just using the regular drug that they did before? [She had had induced labor before.]

R. Yes.

I. Is this the same thing they did before?

R. They didn't have this setup here [she indicated the equipment for infusing the drug], but they used something to induce the labor.

I. Is this the only thing, as far as you know, that is different from the other time?

R. Yes. (#06, black, clinic)

My surprise gave way to the realization that my questionnaire needed some additional items concerning the specific information possessed by a subject, and to the fact that I had some new methodological and ethical problems to deal with.

The new methodological problems were twofold. First, since the questionnaire had been constructed under the unrecognized assumption that research subjects would be aware that they were taking part in research, items that worked perfectly well with aware subjects could be interpreted differently by unaware subjects. Their answers, however, could conceal this fact. To take an example, the question "Can you tell me what you know about the study?" made good sense and elicited useful responses from subjects who knew they were taking part in research. But those who did not know that they were in research responded to the question in various ways. Some thought I was referring to the fact of induction when I mentioned the "study." Others thought I was referring to the machine through which the drug was infused. One subject concluded that I was referring to my own interview. And several presumably had no idea of what I was talking about. However, since such subjects often possessed fragments of knowledge about the study—that a "new drug" was involved, the names of the drugs, or that special monitoring equipment was going to be used—their answers to questions about the study often seemed responsive to my questions.

The second methodological problem stemmed from the fact that unaware subjects could learn from my questions that they were taking part in research, since in order to find out if they knew about the research, I had to mention it. Once they caught on, many unaware subjects answered my original questions as easily as did subjects who knew about the research from the start. Furthermore, unaware subjects had the understandable tendency to cover up their ignorance of something my questions presumed they knew.

It became apparent that I would have to ask subjects *when* they had become aware of the research and if they had learned of it from me. Time and again subjects who had showed awareness of the various elements of the research ended up by telling me that it was I who had clued them in.

Even here there was a problem, however, for before I could ask when they had become aware of the research, I had to be certain that they knew I was talking about the drug study for inducing labor. Where there was any doubt that they knew what I was talking about, I had to provide an explanation of what the research was before I asked them when they became aware of it.

Probably the easiest way to learn what I wanted to know would have been to have asked subjects "Did you know that you are in a research project where there is a 50-50 chance that the drug going into your arm is experimental?" This brings me to the ethical problem raised by my discovery that I was interviewing unaware subjects. At the time of my initial interview, most subjects had been receiving a drug for an hour or two, and were in the early stages of labor. I was in the position of revealing that the drug being used might be experimental. Although I determined that I would have to broach this topic at some point (not necessarily in the initial interview), there were two possible consequences of such a revelation that I was most anxious to avoid.

First, I did not want to alarm subjects as their labor began. Second, I wanted to minimize the probability that subjects would react against the researchers as a result of my activities.

Ways of dealing with these problems emerged as I found that I could be guided by the reaction of subjects to my questions. If I could tell during my first interview (during labor) that a woman did not know about the drug study, I ended the interview immediately. (This did not seem awkward because I had first spent a few minutes on background questions that had nothing to do with the research.) More difficult were the instances in which it appeared that my questions were giving a woman her first realization that she was taking part in a drug study. Whenever this situation arose, I immediately offered a brief, somewhat sugar-coated explanation of the study, leaving it to the follow-up interview to determine just what the woman had understood before the drug infusion had begun. I did not want to frighten subjects in labor. In this explanation I avoided the words "experimental" and "research," as the nurse had instructed. I indicated that there were no risks (rather than no *known* risks), and emphasized the special care they were receiving. To my relief, not one subject gave any indication of becoming alarmed by this explanation, although at least two raised some sharp questions with the research staff after the interview.

I glossed over the aspects that might produce anxiety only in explanations given to subjects in the labor room (first interview) who were obviously in no position to do anything about the anxiety. In cases in which it was during the second interview (after the induction was over) that I found myself explaining the research to subjects, I dropped the sugar coating and explained the research as I understood it. However, I continued to make every effort to defuse any resulting anger toward the researchers. Surprisingly, I found little resentment toward the researchers, and what little there was I dealt with fairly easily. Several women did say, however, that if something had gone wrong with their inductions they might have felt differently about the research.

The following example of this sometimes delicate process of interviewing an unaware subject illustrates many of these problems. We begin in the first interview in the labor room.

I. I understand that one of the things they are doing with your being induced is they might be using a new drug. Did they say anything to you about that?

R. No, they didn't say anything.

I. Did they give you a piece of paper that explained anything about being induced?

R. No.

I. I just want to be sure about this because some of the people having labor induced that I have talked to used a new drug. But they didn't say anything about that or give you a form to sign or anything?

R. No. [pause] I had to sign a form though, but I didn't feel like reading it right then. She told me it was just so they had my agreement to go through with it.

At the second interview, our conversation went as follows:

I. Do you remember yesterday morning, I was asking you about a form? You said you signed one, but you didn't read it?

R. Yes.

I. It was a form that told you that they were using different drugs for inducing labor, and they were comparing . . .

R. Yes, because I asked one of the nurses that was in with me yesterday and I asked her what it was about after I started feeling better. And she was just telling me that they do these experiments with the new drugs and all.

I. OK. So you know about it. That's what I wanted to ask you about, and it would be hard if you hadn't read the paper or they hadn't told you much more.

R. [She laughed] Yes. She explained it to me [during labor].

I. OK. We were talking about yesterday and your nervousness and the nurse giving you the paper. You said you didn't feel like reading it then?

R. No. After she told me they had to have my signature, my agreement, before they could go through with it and that's the only way they could do it, I wanted to go ahead and get it over with, so I decided to go ahead and sign it.

I. Then I came in later and started talking about it and then you started realizing that it was research?

R. Yeah. [laugh] That's when I really thought about what it was.

I. What did you ask the nurse later?

R. When she came back in after we was talking, that's when I was questioning her about it. She was telling me that they were experimenting with new drugs and things. I said how are you all sure that this drug is going to work on me. And she said that this drug would work on me, but they had another one they could give me to seduce [sic] me. (#21, black, clinic)

Thus, because of the factors previously discussed—my desire not to alarm subjects, the fact that unaware subjects easily misinterpreted my questions and responded accordingly, and the fact that they did possess various bits of partial knowledge about the research—I adopted a rather elaborate procedure in interviewing unaware subjects. A carefully presented explanation of the research that would not raise anxiety or hostility toward the researchers had to precede the key questions of when and from whom the subject learned research was taking place. Twenty subjects informed me that I had been the source of that information, and they comprised the group of unaware subjects.

Characteristics of Unaware Subjects.   The likelihood that a subject would be unaware of the research was related to her education, her race, and whether she had a private physician. Not surprisingly, the data in Table 13 indicate that the more dissimilar the subject was from the physicians she saw, the more likely she was to be unaware of the research.

Looking first at the education variable, the critical factor seems to be whether a subject had a high school education. About one-fourth of the subjects with at least a high school education were unaware subjects, compared with the two-thirds of the subjects with less than a high school diploma who were unaware.

A similar finding emerges when private-clinic status is compared. Twenty-two percent of private patients were unaware subjects, while 48 percent of clinic patients were unaware. However, white clinic patients were similar to private patients (all of whom were white); 23 percent of the white

Table 13. Percentage of Unaware Subjects, by Educational Level, by Private-Clinic Status, and by Race (Labor-Induction Study)

Characteristics	Subjects Unaware of Research Before Participation Began	(N)
Education		
Subjects with at least some college	24%	(17)
Subjects with high school diploma	25%	(16)
Subjects with less than high school education	67%	(18)
Private-Clinic Status		
Private patients	22%	(18)
Clinic patients	48%	(33)
Race		
White clinic patients	23%	(13)
Black clinic patients	68%	(19)

clinic patients were unknowing subjects. This means that the private-clinic difference is attributable to the large number of unaware subjects among the black clinic patients. Indeed, 68 percent of the black clinic patients were unaware of the research at the time their participation began.

While numbers are too small to control for education effectively, education and race appear to have independent effects on the probability that a subject would be unaware of the research. None of the 8 private patients with a college degree or more was unaware of the research; 4 of the 9 with less than a college degree were unaware. Furthermore, three of these subjects had the same physician, and, of his six patients in the study, they were the only three who had less than a college degree.

The three unaware white clinic patients present a more confusing picture with regard to education. Two of them came from the group of four white clinic patients with ninth grade education or less; the other was one of the two white clinic patients with some college experience. (No clinic patient had completed college.)

The impact of education was most evident (partially because larger numbers were present) among the black clinic patients. While 4 of 9 black clinic patients with a high school degree or more were unaware of the study, 9 of the 10 black clinic patients with less than a high school degree were unaware of the study.

These findings lend support to the hypothesis that the problem of communicating material necessary to informed consent becomes more serious as the social distance between the physician and the prospective subject increases.* It should be noted again that the responsibility for effective communication failure rests with the physician, not with the subject. If investigators decide to use subjects with low levels of education for procedures that require informed consent, they should recognize that communication problems will be at their maximum and be prepared to accept responsibility for meeting these problems. To pitch a consent form and the explanation that accompanies it to the level of the "average patient" is to risk failing to communicate with those whose education or capacity for understanding is less than average. Such individuals have the right to give informed consent before they are used as research subjects.

The fact that almost 40 percent of the subjects in the labor-induction study participated without knowing about it, even though all procedural requirements for obtaining clearance for the project and informed consent from the subjects were followed, testifies to the need for the investigator to be prepared to communicate at the subject's own level, whatever that level may be.

* None of the doctors involved was black.

Further analysis of the consent problems involved in the study is presented in Chapter Eight.

UNWILLING SUBJECTS

Unwilling subjects knew that research was taking place, but felt constrained to participate. These subjects indicated that they would have preferred not to be in the research; they felt that they had been in a position in which they could not refuse. Four subjects in the labor-induction study were classified as unwilling subjects; two others expressed serious reservations about their own participation. We will examine these important cases individually. No subjects in the starvation-abortion study were classified as unwilling.

The concept of informed consent implies a measure of control by an individual over what is done to him. Individuals classified either as unwilling or unaware subjects clearly lacked such control, but for different reasons. The lack of control of unaware subjects resulted from their lack of knowledge. Control of information is not an uncommon way of controlling a situation, and has been noted before in medical contexts.[7] The lack of control of unwilling subjects was, however, not primarily due to lack of information, but to their doctors' willingness to use the power that derived from the dependency of the patient in the doctor-patient relationship. The reference to the *doctor-patient* relationship rather than to the *researcher-subject* relationship is intentional, because three of the four unwilling subjects were private patients, and it was partly their relationship with their private physician that constrained them in this particular situation.

Although much has been written about doctor-patient relationships, the power dimension is often overlooked, probably because it usually becomes apparent only in situations in which the desires of the doctor and patient diverge. Ordinarily the patient puts himself into the doctor's hands and does what he is told. Indeed, such "cooperative" behavior is part of the expectation of the sick role.[8]

However, dependency is also part of the sick role, and dependency has been shown to be the basis of a power differential in relationships, to the extent that one individual is disproportionately dependent upon the other.[9] The dependency created by the patient's need for help and lack of perceived alternatives to a relationship with the present doctor is well illustrated by excerpts from interviews with unwilling subjects. While the power of the expert was instrumental in the participation of both unaware and unwilling subjects, the latter are distinguished by their awareness and dissatisfaction over having had power exercised at such a crucial time as the birth of a child. Their reactions contained both anger and disappointment.

Excerpts from interviews with the four unwilling subjects are important not only because of what they reveal about the conduct of medical research, but also because of what they reveal about the power and dependency dimensions of the ordinary doctor-patient relationship.

I. Your doctor only said that you would be induced? Did he say anything about new methods or did he just say that they had a drug that was working well?

R. Yes, that's all. Said it's a good chemical. He said Dr. P's [the principal investigator] unit, good chemical, got good nurses, you know.

I. So you came in and they handed you the consent form? The nurses did?

R. Yes. And when I read it I backed off. And my feeling was that I'm not going to be a chemical guinea pig.

I. Then what happened?

R. Then I said I refused to sign it until I see someone who is in charge. Speak to them. And Dr. P spoke to me and from the way, you know, that he spoke it appeared I had no choice, you know, at that point. And then, you know, the nurses sensed that I was a little disturbed by this and one of them brought me an article that was in the newspaper explaining the research in great detail. And I read it. But they were very good, because they gave me information I could accept. And then when you came along with your last question, all of a sudden it dawned on me that it was my doctor's decision that I be in the study.

I. It was your decision, still.

R. No. No. No, I had *no choice*. I'll tell you why. Because my doctor decided I was to be induced. Now the decision of his to induce me and how I was to be induced was his decision. He didn't consult me. He made the decision of what was going to be medically sound for me, and in his medical opinion it was sound for me to be taken care of by these people. So what am I going to do? Say I am going to back out and run away to a different hospital? I mean, it's ridiculous.

I. Perhaps you had the choice of not being in a double-blind drug study, but still using the monitoring equipment and so forth?

R.   No. There was no such choice. It was a package deal.

I.   They do use that monitoring equipment regularly when they have a
case they feel . . .

R.   No. This was not presented to me that I had a choice.

. . .

R.   Right now, I'm not unhappy about it. [This was after the successful
delivery of her baby.] If things had been different I would probably be
complaining. My husband didn't like it when I told him. He didn't like
it at all that they wanted to use me as a guinea pig, you know.

I.   Well, of course, the difficulty is that they eventually have to try things
for the first time on people.

R.   Yeah. But I don't want to be that one.

. . .

I.   If you had decided that you did not want to be in the study, what
would they have done?

R.   I felt that I couldn't not sign. If that makes any sense.

I.   But what would have happened if you *had* refused?

R.   I think Dr. D [her private physician] would have come and given me
hell. (#13, white, private)

This woman felt that since arrangements for her participation in research
had been made by her private physician before she came into the hospital
for her induction, she had no choice but to go along with it, even though
she did not like it. She had not understood about the research aspects of
her induction at the time her physician made the arrangements; she found
out about the research when she was given the consent form in the labor
room. Nevertheless, her description of why she could not refuse at that
point focuses on her relationship with her private physician, and her words
show the inadequacy of conceptions of the doctor-patient relationship as
consensual. "I had no choice . . . because my doctor decided . . ." "Dr. D
would have come and given me hell." She recognized that she was in a

weak position, because, in addition to her status and knowledge disadvantages of which she may or may not have been aware, she was without a viable alternative at that point. "So what am I going to do . . . run away to a different hospital?" Thus, the dependency that resulted from her physical situation as well as her lack of alternatives created the opportunity for the effective exercise of power, which resulted in this subject's unwilling participation in the labor-induction study.

The second unwilling subject was also a private patient, and like the first woman felt that her private physician had given her no choice but to participate. Her description of her experience again highlights the doctor's use of the power that derives both from his control over the patient's knowledge and from the dependency of the patient:

I. How did you find out about the study? You said Dr. D [private physician] told you yesterday that if you wanted to you could?

R. [pause] He almost said, "That's it." [little laugh] "You *are* having . . . [trailed off].

. . .

R. I did not know enough about the drug and what was being done ahead of time. And I am still a little disappointed that I wasn't prepared on Tuesday when I was told about it. I was very disappointed—I won't tell him [her private physician] because I know he would be very upset, because I think he can get that way—but I think that he underestimated my . . . understanding. And this is what upset me most of all. That he told me less because he thought maybe I was . . . [trailed off]. Now, when I had asked a few questions in his office, his reaction was, "No questions. You just go in tomorrow and be a good girl." And I wasn't asking about the baby [about possible complications in delivery]. I wanted to know more about this. And I'll tell you the other thing that really upset me. When I came in and saw I had to sign a release. I didn't know that ahead of time. If I had known I had to sign a release, I might have given it more careful thought. Not that I would have said no. I'm not saying I would not have signed it. But it was thrown at me the minute I walked in. Like am I going to turn around, say forget it, and go home all of a sudden, which I can't do. I *had* to be induced. It showed later that I had to. I just felt that I should have been more informed.

I. The researchers probably assumed your doctor had told you everything, and he assumed they probably would. I don't think anyone is trying to withhold information.

R. No. I have the definite feeling that Dr. D [private physician] was withholding it because it was, you know, "Listen, you don't have to know about it. If I say it's OK, it's OK." Because his attitude was, "Listen, if you were my wife, I'd let her do it, so you can do it," and that's just how he worded it to me. He said to me, "You are not a guinea pig." Even though I said, "You said it's not proved, that it's not on the market." And he said, "Well, you're not a guinea pig. Don't call it an experiment. It's fine."

. . .

I. If you had said you didn't want a new drug, would you have come into the hospital anyway?

R. I don't think I would have had any choice with Dr. D. I think he would have said, "Hey, listen here. Tomorrow is the day and I told you to be ready, and, believe me, it's OK for you." I think I would have had almost no choice. Unless I wanted to say, "Forget it, I'm going to call another doctor." Which I could not do at that point. And I wouldn't anyway.

. . .

I. Why did you agree to participate?

R. I did because I felt I had no choice. That was the main thing.

I. This was what the doctor felt was . . .

R. And I trusted him and his reputation. I knew he was competent and I figured, "Well, he knows what he is doing. OK." And, "I won't go against him," because if I did, I felt that I would have a difficult time. And if I became pregnant again and seeing him, I didn't know how he would treat me as a patient. And that meant more to me. (#24, white, private)

Like the first unwilling subject, this woman felt that her refusal to participate in the labor-induction research would have jeopardized her relationship with her physician (the same in both cases) to the extent that she would need to find another doctor.[10] Since neither of these women wished to find another physician at the time they were ready to go into labor, their physician's power in this situation was substantial. And again the trust in the physician was an important factor, for even though subject #24 felt that she was forced to participate, she still mentioned her trust in her physician and his reputation as an important factor in her participation. Finally, her lack of ease with the situation was heightened by her feeling that she was not informed by her physician as she should have been, a fact that "disappointed" her.

The third unwilling subject was probably the *most unwilling*. Her husband ("H" in the following excerpt from the first interview with this subject) shared her feelings:

I. Why did you participate? [first interview]

H. I don't think they gave us much of a choice.

R. Yeah, really that's true. They asked us if we would sign this thing, and we discussed it.

H. They really didn't give us much of a choice. I think if they had given us more of a choice I think we might have gone a safer route.

R. Yeah.

I. The only other way they could have done it was just to use Pitocin, I guess.

H. Right. Well, she didn't say that. She didn't say we could have Pitocin. I don't know. Maybe I heard her wrong, but that's the impression I got.

R. No, that was my understanding too. [Both the husband and I felt the need to reassure the subject after this exchange]

H. I'm sure Dr. M [private physician] wouldn't subject us to something like this unless it was completely safe. We have a lot of confidence in him.

I. He has had a number of patients induced this way.

H. Yeah, we have a lot of confidence in him, so if he lets it go, I'm sure it's OK. . . .

. . .

I. [second interview] You told me that Dr. M said that you could be induced if you wanted to? He recommended it but he didn't . . .

R. He said there would be a study group which meant that they would monitor the baby's heart and there would be a nurse with me at all times, but he didn't mention any of the drug aspect at all.

I. And then when you came in?

R. She gave me the paper to sign.

I. That was the first you knew about it?

R. Right, that was the first I knew about it.

I. Was your husband with you at that point?

R. No, he was downstairs and I didn't sign it until he came up and I had him read it and we discussed it before we signed it.

I. Was it at all awkward waiting or not?

R. Uh, yes. I found it kind of awkward. I found . . . The thing I found most awkward was that [the research nurse]—she's very nice—but she was in the room and I would have preferred to have discussed it with him privately. I kind of felt we were forced into the situation, you know. If we were alone we maybe wouldn't have made such a rapid decision, you know. We could have been a little bit more open with each other. I just didn't feel quite comfortable discussing it with her.

. . .

I. How did you feel about being asked to participate?

R. I felt uncomfortable about it—I felt very pressured into it. I don't . . . I think maybe if I was aware of it before I came in and Dr. M had explained it to me before, we wouldn't have even hesitated about it, you know. Like you said, we went through all this procedure, and you work yourself up to a point and go in and you can't be too objective. And I felt a great deal of pressure.

. . .

I. If you had decided that you did not want to be in the study, what would they have done?

R. Well, I had the feeling that they would have sent me home by then. That's why we consented. I mean, but they didn't say this, you know. It was just sort of overall atmosphere or something. Sort of intuitive type of thing. Which probably . . . which was wrong, you know, but this is the way we both felt.

. . .

I. Why did you agree to participate?

R. Well, one of the main reasons was we found out that Dr. M was aware of it. We felt that he wouldn't subject me to anything that wasn't safe. And the other reason, the other main reason, I think is we felt we didn't have much of a choice and therefore I'd be going home and I didn't want this. I was in here and I had gone through two sleepless nights and I wasn't about to go home.

. . .

I. Did you believe that being in this research (or refusing to participate) might affect the care you would receive or the way you were treated while in the hospital?

R. Yes.

I. In what way?

R. In a negative way if I refused.

I. Specifically how?

R. Um . . . well . . .

I. That you might be sent home or in another way?

R. Either that, or they might be annoyed because we didn't do it, and
therefore, in some way, not give me the attention that I would require.
(#45, white, private)

This subject stressed the pressure that arose from learning about the
research in the labor room, rather than direct pressure from her physician.
Like the first two women, she felt that a decision to refuse would have
meant she would be sent home, not an attractive option for a woman who
has prepared herself for childbirth. However, the pressure that resulted in
this woman's becoming an unwilling subject was also a result of a situation
created by a private physician, in this case his failure to inform his patient
that he was putting her into a program that involved an experimental drug.
That a doctor was willing to take such action is evidence of the extent to
which doctors can become accustomed to assuming control over the fate of
patients; thus, the doctor-patient relationship is sometimes analogized to a
parent-child relationship.[11] That this assumption of control can go beyond
the degree desired by the patient is demonstrated by the unwilling subjects
in the labor-induction study.

The last unwilling subject was the only clinic patient of the four. She was
a highly educated Puerto Rican woman whose husband was in graduate
school. The husband was present during the interview, and his translations
and comments are included (as "H") in the excerpts quoted below.

I. You told me yesterday that all you knew about the research before it
started was what you read on the paper? That was all?

R. Yes.

H. They told her, "Just read this and sign."

R. No. No. No "read." Just "Sign here."

H. "Sign here." Just "Sign here." Then, when I came in she [his wife]
told me, "They made me . . . uh . . . I signed a paper that said they are
going to experiment with me, and this and this," and I told her, "Why
did you sign it?" There wasn't any alternative. They don't give you an
alternative.

I. Did you two discuss it at all?

H. No, because I was downstairs at the registration office making all the papers, and she was alone upstairs with the nurse, and that was when she signed the paper. I didn't even read it. I didn't even see the paper. [He told me he had looked for the paper after he arrived, but could not find it.]

   . . .

H. [translating] She didn't want to be a means to an experiment. To be used in an experiment.

R. Yes, because in the clinic they use you too much to make experiment with the students. For example, some doctors come and see you and another doctor [will then] see you and maybe say the same thing and ask the same questions. Oh! When you are finished you are tired of everything.

I. But you understood when they gave you the paper that they were going to be using a new drug? That it was experimental?

R. No, not when she gave me the paper, but when I sign something I always read it first. (#15, Puerto Rican, clinic)

In this case, being in the labor room in the belief that induction was necessary, being somewhat anxious about the delivery and eager to have it over with, and being unaware of any alternative to participating in the study combined to cause this woman to agree to participate although she did not want to be in a research study. Of the four subjects, she was the least unwilling, however.

Discussion.   Unwilling subjects were easily the most highly educated of the types of subjects. Of the four labor-induction subjects who had graduate degrees, three were unwilling subjects. The fourth unwilling subject had three years of college. Three were private patients; the fourth had used the hospital's clinics because of her husband's connection with the university as a postdoctoral fellow.

How is it that four highly educated, high status women became unwilling subjects? The answer lies in the way they learned about the research, their awareness that risks would be present if an experimental drug was involved, and their lack (for several reasons) of a viable alternative to participating. Let us briefly examine each of these factors.

First, none of the four knew before she reached the labor room that an experimental drug might be used, although, with the exception of the Puerto Rican woman who came through the clinic, all had been informed by their physicians that they were to be "study patients." What this involved had not been specified to them.

Second, the impact of their learning of the experimental drug in the labor room was heightened by these women's high degree of education. Highly educated persons were most likely to be familiar with research in general, and to be aware that risks could be present. These subjects all showed some sensitivity to the issue of risk:

H. It's curious that there was no explanation about the consequences of that drug. Right now, I don't have any idea of what can be the consequences of it. (#15, Puerto Rican, clinic)

R. I know about new drugs. So I didn't want to sign. (#13, white, private)

R. I thought, "I might as well get it over with. As long as this isn't dangerous, then OK." (#24, white, private)

R. Well, the thing we were really most concerned with was, you know, when you think of research . . . and it did have down [on the consent form] that any new drug could be dangerous—they don't know the effects of it—this is kind of . . . you know . . . you start thinking all sorts of things. (#45, white, private)

We mentioned that of the four subjects with graduate degrees, three were unwilling subjects. The fourth subject with a graduate degree, whose case will be discussed shortly, also had many characteristics of an unwilling subject, including concern over the possibility of unknown risks. As she noted:

R. It's the drug. The word "drug." The connotation "drug." Especially after Thalidomide and things like that. I mean, you read about these articles and then it's too late, you know. So that . . . well, I didn't even take an aspirin all through my pregnancy. That's what I mean. For 9 months if I had a pain, I stuck with it. That's why I said that it was very . . . almost amusing that I found myself in this particular situation and this whole thing was slowly revealed to me, because I know I would have said no if given time to think about it. And

I feel that I should have been told the day before that there was a drug. (#19, white, private)

Highly educated subjects were, therefore, aware of what was potentially involved in the administration of an experimental drug. Furthermore, these high status women may have been more willing to raise question that might seem to imply skepticism about physicians. However, it was ultimately their faith in their physicians as well their dependency and lack of awareness of alternatives to participation that appear to have led them to go ahead, however unhappy they were about it.

The third element that combined with the two just mentioned was not seeing a reasonable alternative to going ahead once they found out what was involved. None thought they had any choice, either because they believed that their condition dictated that they be induced, because they were mentally committed to going ahead (they were, after all, in the labor room and admitted to the hospital, and had made arrangements for their other children), or because they thought that backing out would mean that they would have to sever or threaten their relationship with the obstetrician they had seen throughout their pregnancy.

Thus, unwilling subjects were created by informing educated women (who understood that risks could be involved) of the research in such a way or at such a time that they felt they had no alternative to participation.

The response of two other women—both of whom were classed as benefiting subjects—exhibited the same pattern of disquiet about the research. However, since both of these women recognized that they had the choice of waiting, they were not classified as unwilling. Nevertheless, their cases were strikingly similar to those just discussed. Both were highly educated private patients, both knew before they came in that they were to be "study patients," but neither knew an experimental drug was to be involved. Both had reservations about participating and raised many questions. For example, one asked her husband for advice, a practice she described as unusual for her:

R. She [the nurse] gave me the form and at that point I had a little bit of reservation. When my husband came up—although a decision like that is usually left up to me in our relationship—I felt that I wanted somebody else to make the decision for me, that I didn't want the full responsibility because I felt a little bit of reservation at that point when I realized that I might be getting a drug that wasn't completely tested at that point. (#46, white, private)

Both of these women indicated that they might not have participated if they

had known before they came to the hospital that an experimental drug
might be used:

R. I just knew I was going to be part of a study group, and I was told that
all it would mean was that the baby's heartbeat was going to be monitored. I didn't know anything about a new drug. As I said yesterday, I
might have reconsidered because I am one who reads articles about
people in experiments and say "Well, they shouldn't have been in an
experiment, anyway." I'm very conservative in that way. Not
politically, but in that way. (#19, white, private)

I. Would it have made any difference, do you think, if you had known
about it before you came in?

R. Yes, it might have. I think we would probably have been more in conflict. Dualistic, that's the word. I would have been more nervous about
it.* (#46, white, private)

One reason why neither of these women was classified as unwilling was
that they expressed some awareness of alternatives to participation and
chose the research over these alternatives. The alternatives were not attractive, however, since a heavy commitment to induction had been made
by being admitted to the hospital, and the alternative would have been to
leave. In their own words, they describe their alternatives:

R. Oh, I think that once I had read that thing, if I had said to them, "I
didn't realize that there would be any risk involved; I assumed the
standard Pitocin would be used and I would rather not partake," I
think . . . I know they would have let me go. I mean, I would have
been embarrassed, but they wouldn't have kept me here. (#46, white,
private)

R. I wasn't that desperate to get in. I wanted to be with Dr. M [private phy-
sician] and he induces on Wednesday, so it was this Wednesday or I

---

* This comment again raises the issue of whether the disclosure of risks necessary to informed
consent may cause undesirable anxiety among some patients. This issue is difficult because of
the very real possibility that an investigator might justify his witholding information that might
cause subjects to decline on the grounds of not wanting to make them anxious. This is the sort of
conflict of interest problem for which such bodies as review committees are useful.

would have to wait until next Wednesday. Otherwise I could have gone in tomorrow [Friday] with Dr. R [another physician in the group practice]. (#19, white, private)

It could be reasonably argued that the alternative of leaving the hospital was not a very genuine one once they had already been admitted to the hospital. In fact, one of these women had been extremely worried about her delivery (she had lost a baby late in pregnancy) and had been most eager to have the baby at the earliest possible moment, by whatever means. The other woman told me of having made arrangements for the care of her son while she was hospitalized. A change of mind *would* have been awkward and would have caused unknown difficulties.

Ultimately, the reason these two were not classified as unwilling was because they showed awareness of alternatives, and because they gave a *positive* reason when asked why they agreed to participate.

I. Why did you agree to participate?

R. Again, I have to say it was a completely selfish reason, that I was concerned about the safety of the baby and wanted the baby to come. (#46, white, private)

I. What sorts of things did you ask questions about?

R. Well, I wanted to know how relatively safe it was, how long it had been used, would it have any effects on the baby?

I. And they satisfied you on all of those things?

R. Well, enough to continue. I didn't feel like turning around and going home at that point. (#19, white, private)

In addition to the six subjects discussed above, at least four *unaware* subjects gave explicit indications that they might not have been willing to participate if they had understood the project.

R. I think if my doctor had said, "We are debating on using a new drug that hasn't been proven yet but is in the experimental stage," I would have said, "Forget it." (#29, white, private)

I. If you had known it was research, do you think you would have agreed to come in or do you think you would have waited?

R. I might not have.

I. You think it might have made a difference?

R. Yeah. (#50, black, clinic)

I. What would you have done if you had had time to think about it this time?

R. I think I would have been unwilling, say, if I had known about it a month beforehand. And I had really thought about it. But it turned out very satisfactory. (#27, white, private)

I. What if they had explained everything before they started this time? Did you say you probably wouldn't have done it?

R. Yeah, I probably wouldn't. (#21, black, clinic)

It is possible that others among the unaware subjects would have given similar responses. Subjects were not questioned systematically on this point, since the existence of unaware subjects was not anticipated at the time the questionnaire was drawn up.

BENEFITING SUBJECTS

Those I call "benefiting subjects" participated knowingly (although there was great variation in knowledge) and voluntarily (although not free from a variety of pressures). They participated primarily because they felt that it was to their benefit to do so. The benefit was often convenience, although some medical benefits were also mentioned. The perceived benefits were not always real, but belief in them was real and was the stated reason for these subjects' participation. Twenty-two of the 51 labor-induction subjects (43 percent) were classified as benefiting subjects, as were 5 of the 7 starvation-abortion subjects.

In both studies, participation in the research project effectively hastened an event that the women were most eager to have take place. Not one subject in the labor-induction study said that she would liked to have waited longer before having her baby (although two or three expressed a preference for having it "naturally" rather than by induction). Perhaps the most frequently made comment from the labor-induction subjects concerned their overwhelming impatience with being pregnant and their readiness to deliver. Thirteen benefiting subjects in the labor-induction study gave such responses as the *major* reason they had agreed to be research subjects, though this was expressed in various ways.

I. Why did you decide to participate?

R. Just to get it over and done with. He said the baby was all formed and everything, so why be uncomfortable? (#41, white, clinic)

I. Why did you decide to participate?

R. Because if they thought I was ready, why should I go on a couple more days when I felt uncomfortable? I was getting a lot of pressure [from the baby] . . . (#08, white clinic)

I. Why did you decide to participate? [long pause] Was it just because your doctor thought it best?

R. No, because he didn't. He gave us a choice. He said I could wait because I was only 2 or 3 more days, or I could come and have it done. I guess for the very personal reason that I was getting tired of carrying myself around. (#22, white, private)

R. He said he thought he could get me admitted as a study patient. He thought that was the only way he could get me in today. He said I was ready. I was a week overdue and I had been very uncomfortable and having contractions on and off. (#19, white, private)

R. Because I was anxious to have the baby fast. I have to say it was a completely selfish reason, that I was concerned about the safety of the baby and wanted the baby to come. And then, of course, because I'm not adverse to . . . you know, helping further educational purposes. That was secondary, but certainly wasn't the primary reason. (#46, white, private)

I. Why do you think your doctor asked if you wanted to be a subject in this research?

R. Maybe because I was late, impatient, uncomfortable, nervous, couldn't wait. [laughed]

I. Why did you agree to participate?

R. Same reason. Nervous, impatient. (#12, white, private)

R. Well, I had been so late and I was afraid that the baby was going to keep gaining weight and gaining weight. I know I wouldn't have been induced in any other way. At least I don't think so. I mean, there was no chance of any other way of going in but this way. (#40, white, private)

R. I was 3 weeks late. They couldn't let it go longer. And he said it wouldn't harm me or the baby—said it was safe. They know what they are doing. And if there is anything I can help them out with, great. As long as it didn't endanger me or the baby, what should I say about it? (#11, white, clinic)

Some of these women were probably giving reasons why they had agreed to have labor induced rather than why they had decided to take part in research. As we have seen, many women confused the nonresearch with the research aspects of their induction, and were unable to separate them for purposes of my interviews. Also, in many cases subjects' decisions to have labor induced were made before they knew that research was to be involved. Thus, in a real sense, the reason why some women participated in the research was because they had already decided to have labor induced, and this was merely how the physicians proposed to accomplish it.

The above quotations show that some subjects had more than one reason for participating. However, all of this group of subjects indicated that the *primary* reason was that the research was the quickest route to the delivery room, and they wanted to have their babies as soon as possible. In some cases this was because of their own discomfort or impatience; in other cases they were eager to have their baby at the earliest possible time because they believed it was to their baby's benefit to do so.

Eagerness to get into the hospital was even a stronger motivation factor for subjects in the starvation-abortion study. It was the major reason for participation given by 4 of the 7 subjects in that study (compared to 13 of 51 in the labor-induction study). Once they had decided to have an abortion they understandably wanted the decision carried out as soon as possible. In addition, the subjects in the starvation study had each been approved for an abortion through the hospital's regular procedures, and had been told that they would be called when the hospital had room for them. They had been waiting for varying lengths of time, some for several weeks. All of them knew that the hospital would not give a saline injection after the twentieth week of pregnancy. As that time approached, they became more anxious.

R. Well, it was so close to time, to the 20 weeks. I and my husband wanted everything before the 20 weeks . . . to hurry up and have everything done.

I. Were you afraid that they wouldn't call you or something might happen or what?

R. They said that they didn't have too many beds, you know, and the first chance that they called me I decided I would come on in. (#63, black)

Eagerness to have the procedure over with was also the primary motive for both of the following, who put their reasons for participating very concisely:

R. The main thing was just to get it over with. (#65, black)

R. Because I figured this was the earliest date I could get into the hospital and get out. (#67, black)

One starvation-abortion subject whose reason for participating had to be repeatedly modified as she learned more about the research had originally agreed to participate because she believed that the research was her earliest ticket into the hospital. Her case was mentioned at the end of Chapter Four. She had been called by a member of the research team and asked to participate. She agreed because of her eagerness to get into the hospital. Shortly thereafter she learned that she had been scheduled for admission that day without being in the research. On learning this, she gave the matter further thought. She decided to go ahead with the research for two reasons. First, she understood (incorrectly) that the research would pick up her entire hospital bill. Second, she gave the research requirements some thought and decided that "losing the weight and having the blood tests might not be so bad after all, maybe. I hadn't had any [blood tests] for a long time and had forgotten what it was like. I thought [the fast] wouldn't be so bad for three days" (#102, black).

When the fast was well underway she found out about her misunderstanding of the financial aspect; furthermore "I couldn't take being this hungry and everything. I thought I might as well get transferred to [the regular floor] and get it over with since I had to pay a bill anyway." At this point, to her consternation, "They told me that they couldn't transfer me over there because of the bed space, that they would have to send me home and I would have to wait for a call to get in. So I just stuck it out." This story had a somewhat happier end than it might have. The subject was able to use her sullen anger about the circumstances just described and the researchers' guilt over the series of misunderstandings to win some concessions from the researchers. She said that they agreed to halve the number of blood tests she would have to undergo and to allow her more tea and coffee.

Furthermore, in the negotiations that went on, the investigators took the time to discuss with her the purpose of the research, the problems in which the researchers were interested, and the groups that would perhaps benefit from the research. She recognized that research into the effects of malnutrition on the unborn would have importance for poverty stricken mothers, and ended up feeling that her contribution to the research was most worthwhile. I believe that if she had been approached in these terms from the beginning that she would have willingly participated, because of the poverty in her own background.

This case was easily the most complex from the standpoint of reasons for participation. The subject began as a poorly informed, benefiting subject, and ended up as a committed subject.

In addition to the labor-induction subjects who participated because the study represented the quickest route into the hospital, there were other types of benefiting subjects. Three subjects gave as their primary reason for agreeing to participate the fact that being in the study would allow them the convenience of planning and knowing ahead of time when they would be admitted. Two of these women lived more than a hour from the hospital and had a history of fast labors.

Convenience was also the major factor for the physician's wife, mentioned earlier, who came into the hospital in labor only to have her labor stop. Her own physician, who had assigned patients to the study, checked and found out that there was a research spot open that day. She told me, "We thought I was in labor and then it stopped and he was going to send me home. Then he said I could go on this study, I could have the baby now" (#32, white, private). The benefit to her from participating was most clear, and, as she said, "I didn't think of it so much as an experiment as much as a case of just being induced and getting it over with."

The third type of benefit mentioned was medical benefit. Three of the five who participated for medical benefit did so because they believed that the "new drug" was better. This was, of course, the research question to which an answer was not yet available. Why these women thought they were getting a better drug is not clear, but this belief was an important reason why they agreed to participate:

R. Well, from what I have read about it it's just a little bit different—it's supposedly stronger than the drug they had used previously. I did it because they assured me that it would be best for me, and I wanted what was best for me and my baby. (#17, black, clinic)

R. They tell me that this works better than the old drug, so . . . [pause] I'll let you know on the second interview.

I. Why did you decide to participate?

R. I don't know . . . simply because they told me it would work better than the "pit." You know, the other drug. That's all. [pause] I believe them. (#02, white, clinic)

R. [I did it] just to get it over with. And if the research drug was used, it would be quicker, I suppose. The only personal benefit to me was to make it easier. (#03, white, private)

The other two labor-induction subjects who gave medical benefit as the reason for their participation referred to the special attention, the constant presence of the research nurses, and the routine use of the fetal monitoring equipment as major factors in their decision to participate. Even in these cases the eagerness of the women to have their babies may have been as important or more important than the medical benefit; in any event they were classified as benefiting subjects.

I. Why did you agree to participate?

R. I wanted to have a baby. See, this study was very minor. I was told that it was a great opportunity, that it was better that I be in the study instead of being normally induced because of the nurses and supervision. (#49, white, private)

R. I agreed because I felt that I was going to be induced in any case, and it was choice of coming in with the regular induction or coming in with this. And being advised that this was really superior.

H.* . . . if she came in today, she could be induced under this drug study and there would be a team of people who would carefully supervise her, whereas if she came in on the weekend they wouldn't be here. He left the decision to us, but we could tell . . . I mean, he sort of recommended that we come in. (#34, white, private)

Only the fifth benefiting subject in the starvation-abortion study has not been discussed. Just as there were three subjects in the labor-induction study who participated at least partially because of nonexistent benefits (the assumed superiority of the experimental drug), one starvation-abortion subject cited a nonexistent benefit for her participation. Although she was aware of the research, she apparently decided that since *physicians* were starving her there must be a *medical reason* as well and that being starved would help the abortion (see Chapter Four). The confusion of subject and patient roles evidenced by this woman was rather common, and is one of the barriers to informed consent discussed in Chapter Eight.

Characteristics of Benefiting Subjects. Many subjects in both studies agreed to participate in research for the nonaltruistic reason that they believed that it was to their benefit (convenience or medical) to do so. What were the characteristics of these subjects, and how did they differ from other subjects? Part of the answer is contained in Table 14.

More than half of the subjects who had at least a high school education gave personal benefit as the major reason for their participation, whereas only 3 of the 18 subjects with less than a high school degree gave such a reason. The private-clinic comparison shows a similar difference. While 56 percent of the private patients were benefiting subjects, 36 percent of the clinic patients gave personal benefit as their reason for agreeing to take part. However, this difference was completely due to a racial difference among the clinic patients—among white clinic patients the percentage of benefiting subjects was similar to the rate among private patients. Very few (4 of 19) black clinic patients participated because of the benefits they perceived.

Since unknowing subjects made up the majority of subjects other than those in the benefiting category, the differences among these categories are

* Respondent's husband

Table 14.   Percentage of Benefiting Subjects by Educational Level, by Private-Clinic Status, and by Race (Labor-Induction Study)

Characteristics	Benefiting Subjects	(N)
Education		
Subjects with at least some college	53%	17
Subjects with high school diploma	62%	16
Subjects with less than high school education	17%	18
Private-Clinic Status		
Private patients	56%	18
Clinic patients	36%	33
Race		
White clinic patients	62%	13
Black clinic patients	21%	19

reduced when we consider the reasons for participation only of those who actually were aware of the research. The differences along the private-clinic and racial dimensions shrink to nothing when we consider only subjects who knew of the research before their involvement began.* Thus, of the patients who had the opportunity to have a reason for participation—that is, among those who knew they were subjects—the major variables fail to distinguish among them with regard to the importance of personal benefit as a motivating factor. About three out of every four knowing subjects gave this as their main reason for participating.

One variable may help explain the differences in types of subjects. Benefiting subjects were more likely than other *knowing* subjects to have known about the research before they were admitted to the hospital, al-

* Among the subjects who knew of the research before their participation began, 9 of 13 (69 percent) of the college educated subjects, 10 of 12 (83 percent) of the high school graduates, and 3 of 6 (50 percent) of those with less than a high school diploma were benefiting subjects. Of the private patients 10 of 14 (71 percent) were benefiting as were 8 of 10 (80 percent) white clinic patients and 4 of 6 (67 percent) of the black clinic patients. The overall average for clinic patients was identical to that of private patients, 71 percent (12 of 17).

though the difference was not a large one. It makes sense that subjects who had more time to consider a decision would be more likely to give thought to the research's advantages to themselves. Low educated subjects who did not learn of the research until in the labor room were likely to end up as indifferent subjects. High educated subjects who learned of the research in the labor room were, as was already pointed out, the pool from which the unwilling subjects were drawn. Perhaps if subjects in both of these latter groups had been given information and time to make a decision before they were admitted, most of them would have ended up either as benefiting subjects or as committed subjects.

INDIFFERENT SUBJECTS

Indifferent subjects expressed no interest in the research and gave only one reason for participating—that it was what the doctors wanted. They seemed to have made no decision to participate; they could mention no factors that they had weighed in their decision. They had apparently simply gone along with a sequence of events as it developed. Indifferent subjects showed under questioning that they were aware that research was taking place, but their stated reason for participation gave no indication of this awareness. In other words, their stated reasons for participation were no different from the stated reasons of unaware subjects.

Three labor-induction subjects were classified as indifferent subjects. No starvation-abortion subjects were so classified. Subjects were classified as indifferent mainly on the basis of their responses to questions about why they agreed and the factors they considered.

I. Did they say anything about using a new drug?

R. Yeah, they said something about that this morning. That's the first thing they said. They told me they had an old one and a new one and she didn't say which one they were going to use.

I. Do you know why they didn't say? Did they explain that?

R. No. She didn't really say why. It's an experience [sic] or something to find out which one works the best.

I. Why did you decide to participate?

R. I don't know. How do I explain this? He wanted to know if I wanted to have my baby today, and I told him yes. So he said they would induce labor and I said, "Yeah, uh-huh." 'Cause I'm ready to get it over with. That's the reason I said yes. (#28, black, clinic)

I. What did he say when he told you about being induced?

R. He said I could be induced if I wanted. As a matter of fact, he said I didn't have too much choice because I was 2 weeks overdue. So he told me it would be best to go ahead and induce labor instead of just letting me sit around and try to get going on my own.

I. I'd like to know what you knew or understood about the study yesterday.

R. Well, I knew it was supposed to stop my pains and everything. And the doctor said it was supposed to make it easier to have the baby. He said it might be a little uncomfortable, that the pains might be hard. And they *were* harder. And that it would be a lot quicker than having it on my own natural labor pains. I guess that's about it.

I. Why did you agree to participate?

R. Just to have the baby. (#25, black, clinic)

I. Why did you decide to participate?

R. Just because I am late. I should have had the baby the thirteenth.

I. Was there any particular reason you wanted to be in research study, or did you?

R. No. I just wanted to have the baby.

. . .

I. Could you describe how you were told about the research and how the doctor asked you to participate?

R. Dr. S [house staff] told me about the research, you know, about being induced and everything. And at the time I went along with everything, because I figured I was late, and I wanted to get it done and over with.

I. He mentioned that they were using a new drug?

R. Uh . . . I didn't know anything about the new drug or anything until I got to the hospital, and then Dr. P [principal investigator] explained the new drug and everything and what it would do.

I. Did Dr. S tell you there was research to it or did he just talk about being induced?

R. Just about being induced. Not particularly about it being a research project or anything.

. . .

I. Why did you agree to participate?

R. Because I wanted to have the baby and I figured I was late. (#14, white, clinic)

Several elements common to these three subjects define their indifference to the research and help to account for it as well. All of these elements were present in at least some other subjects, but the particular cluster of factors was characteristic only of the indifferent group.

Indifferent subjects had low levels of education (one had a high school degree, the other two did not), and became aware of the research in the labor room after their admission to the hospital. As already pointed out, most poorly educated subjects who did not know of the research before they were admitted ended up as unaware subjects; the best educated subjects who did not know of the research before admission tended to become unwilling subjects. Learning of the research for the first time after admission to the hospital, then, was of great importance for the extent of awareness of the research and for the degree to which the subject was able to make a free decision.

The three indifferent subjects also gave several indications of confusing the induction itself with the research. Without the direction provided by the interviews, these subjects, like some others, probably could have made no separation. Thus, their decision to go along with having their labor induced was the only decision they made. When they reached the hospital, they learned more about how this was going to be done, but they gave no indications of making a second decision. The decision had apparently already been made. Hence, when I asked why they had agreed to participate in the research, these subjects could only give me the reasons why they needed to have labor induced.

Parenthetically, I would also like to note that an indifferent subject may not fit the definition of volunteer as it is sometimes construed. T. F. Fox, for example, argues that the word "volunteer" implies far more than passive participation—one reason why a journal reference to "a group of volunteer mice" would seem odd.[12]

COMMITTED SUBJECTS

Committed subjects agreed primarily because they wanted to help the researchers or make a contribution to medical progress. They may have had additional reasons for agreeing, but they gave this as the most important reason. Some other subjects apparently developed a commitment to the research while actually participating in it, but this typology is based on pre-participation motivations.

I did not find many committed subjects. Only 2 of the 51 labor-induction subjects were classified as committed subjects; 2 of the 7 starvation-abortion subjects were so classified. There was an interesting contrast, however, in the basis for commitment in the two studies.

Although the commitment did not seem to be intense in the labor-induction study, participation did seem to be totally altruistic for these two subjects. We now examine these cases in some detail.

I. Could you tell me a little about the study—what's it all about?

R. Well, from what I understand they are using a blind method of induction. And they are trying three different types of induction to see which is the most effective . . . which has the least effects . . . aftereffects. Which to me is great.

I. Why?

R. Because the better methods they come up with the better off women will be.

I. And you are glad to help?

R. Sure, because labors are not the most pleasant things in the world, so if there is anything they can come up with that makes it a little easier or a little safer . . .

. . .

I. Why did you agree to participate?

R. No particular reason. I just . . . I go along with research. I think research is the best method of perfecting something. You certainly can't
perfect it without the research.

I. But a lot of people think, "Let them perfect it on somebody else."

R. No. As I said before, when they finally do get around to using this in a
hospital like this, it's already been just about as tested as it's going to
get. This is more or less practical research, to see the more practical
and most effective. In respect to safety and everything, I would
imagine that it was as safe as it could possibly be.

I. Are you assuming that or did they say so?

R. I'm assuming this would probably be it. Since they are people in the
medical profession and are interested in saving life, not taking it away.
I would imagine they wouldn't do anything or use any drugs that
would be known to have ill effects.

I. Were there any other factors you considered in your decision?
Anything you wanted to know more about before you agreed?

R. I had agreed before I actually asked any more questions. It was sufficient to me that this would benefit people. And being a mother and
having had labor before, I would very definitely wish the best way
possible and the quickest way possible to be used. And if this would
help other new mothers, that's good enough for me. (#30, white, clinic)

This subject indicated at both interviews that the desire to help other
people was her primary motivation. It was the first reason she mentioned
when asked why she agreed. There were obviously other factors in her decision; in the quote above she mentioned her belief that risks were minimal.
This assumption was based on her high faith in the medical profession
rather than on specific information. Elsewhere she said that she had
expressed a general preference for being induced to the physicians at the
clinic some weeks before they asked her if she wanted to participate. But
her *primary* reason for participation, in contrast to the other 49 subjects we
have discussed, was to help the researchers find a better way to induce
labor. She mentioned her own previous experience in having babies (she
had three) as contributing to her feeling on this matter.

The other committed subject in the labor-induction study probably had had the most extensive prior experience with research into problems of pregnancy and became involved in the present study in perhaps the most unusual way. The patient of one of the faculty members of the medical school, she had been referred to him by her own obstetrician in a city more than 2 hours distant because she required intrauterine blood tranfusions due to an Rh problem with her baby. She was highly aware of the unanswered questions in pregnancy and had been the beneficiary of very recent advances; she had been involved in procedures that were still experimental throughout the latter part of a difficult pregnancy.

As described earlier, she became invôlved in the study through some chance factors. She had been admitted to the hospital the afternoon before her induction, and was in the final stages of preparation for labor-induction on a morning when the researchers found out that their scheduled subject had already gone into labor and would not need induction. The principal investigator learned that this woman was already on the floor and was being prepared for induction. He approached her physician to see if he would agree to her participation. Both he and she agreed, and the randomized study medication was substituted for the drug she was ready to receive.

I. How did you feel about being asked to participate?

R. I just felt that maybe it would help somebody learn something.

I. It didn't upset you though?

R. No.

I. Were you pleased about the research, or did you not care too much one way or the other?

R. I think I was pleased in a way.

. . .

I. Why did you agree to participate? What reasons did you give yourself?

R. Just for research, I guess. To help somebody.

I. Did you consider any other things?

R. No. (#48, white, faculty patient)

This subject was one of the least educated of all subjects (eighth grade) and had only a fair understanding of the research (she didn't understand, for example, that more than one drug was involved or that it was a double-blind study). It seems to be a reasonable speculation that the difficulties with her pregnancy and previous experience with research were the key factors in her altruistic response.

Three other labor-induction subjects mentioned benefit to others as a factor in their decision in response to the open-ended questions about reasons for participation. These subjects were not classified as committed subjects for two different reasons.

First, one subject explicitly stated that the altruistic motive was secondary.

I.   Why did you decide to participate?

R.   Because I was anxious to have the baby fast. With no complications or with as few complications as possible. Also . . . I mean, secondary was the fact of experimenting with all this stuff. 'Cause they really don't know much about labor—that comes back to my complications again with labor and contractions. But it was mainly a selfish reason. (#46, white, private)

The stated link between having had difficulties in pregnancy and considering the benefits to others of participating should again be noted. This subject was classified as a benefiting subject because personal benefit was the primary reason for her participation.

Second, two subjects who spontaneously mentioned altruistic motivations did so only in the *second* interview, after the research and their delivery had been completed, and after they had had considerable opportunity to learn about the research and its scientific importance. In the first interview their stated reasons for participation were quite different:

I.   [first interview] Why did you decide to participate?

R.   Well, I'm 3 weeks late and he said it wouldn't harm me or the baby—said it was safe. They know what they are doing.

         . . .

I.   [second interview] Why did you agree to participate?

R.   Well, I had confidence in the doctor; I knew that he wasn't going to give me anything to hurt me. And if there is anything I can help them out with, great. And as long as it didn't endanger me or the baby, what should I say about it? (#11, white, clinic)

I. [first interview] Why did you decide to participate?

R. I don't know. How do I explain this? He wanted to know if I wanted to have my baby today, and I told him yes. So he said they would induce labor and I said, "Yeah, un-huh." 'Cause I'm ready to get it over with. That's the reason I said yes.

. . .

I. [second interview] Why did you agree to participate?

R. Well, let me see. One reason was that maybe my experience might lead to some improvement of medical science.

I. That was the main reason for you?

R. Yes.

I. What factors did you consider? Anything else?

R. That was pretty much it. (#28, black, clinic)

Since postparticipation answers may have reflected things learned about or reflected on while *participating* rather than while *deciding* to participate, the answer given at the first interview was assumed to be a more accurate indication of subjects' original reasons for participating. (Indeed, an important reason for doing two interviews with labor-induction subjects was to uncover this type of situation, which could have been misleading if subjects were only interviewed after their participation was completed.) Thus, these two cases (like all others) were classified on the basis of their first responses; the first case as a benefiting subject, the second as an indifferent subject. This last case, incidentally, illustrates an opportunity for developing in subjects a commitment to research that can be lost if the research is not presented carefully to subjects. This lost educational opportunity is discussed again later.

Although small numbers require this to be only suggestive, highly educated subjects tended not to mention benefit to science as a reason for their participation. This is true even though they were the most articulate and gave the most detailed responses. Of subjects who knew of the research, 1 of 13 with at least some college spontaneously mentioned benefit to science, as did 2 of 12 with high school degrees and 2 of 6 with less than high school education. This, incidently, is consistent with the results of a study by Martin et al. of people's willingness to participate in four hypothetical projects of varying risks.[13] In the four groups compared, it was found that prisoners were most willing to volunteer, followed by low-income persons, firemen and policemen, and professional persons. The differences among these groups were most pronounced where the risk was highest.

The explanation for this is not clear. Martin et al. found that their professional respondents were the only group that did not emphasize the theme of "human responsibility."[14] It also seems likely that appreciation of the risks of medical research is positively associated with education. And it may also be that high status patients assume that low status patients will be used for research purposes, as they have been traditionally used for teaching purposes. This could make it increasingly difficult to recruit research subjects as the growth of third party payment for medical care, particularly by the government, reduces further the population of ward patients, and as sophistication about medical matters increases in the general population. Although this class variation is not well documented at this point, it is of sufficient importance to merit future study.

Turning to the starvation-abortion study, a different and interesting factor was involved in the cases of the two committed subjects—their Catholicism. For both Catholic women, benefit to others was cited as their most important reason for participation.

I.   Why did you agree to participate?

R.   Because of the good benefits I think will come of it.

I.   To whom?

R.   Well, to other people. (#106, white)

I.   Why did you agree to participate?

R.   I liked the idea [of the research] and I wanted to come into the hospital as soon as I could . . . I could be a part of the advancement of medical science, plus it would be a comfort to me. (#101, white)

In the latter quote, reference is made to the interesting aspect of these two Catholic's reasons for participation. Both felt that research participation could add a "positive aspect" to what they saw as an essentially negative experience. Both had moral reservations concerning abortion and feared that they were committing an excessively selfish act in having an abortion. (One was unmarried, the other desired to maintain her present family size.) The opportunity to participate in research and perhaps to help future babies was seen as a counterbalance to negative feelings about their own abortion decisions.

Interesting also was the fact that both of these women mentioned their opportunity to be of service to others in response to questions concerning whether they received *personal* benefit from participating. In addition to mentioning the usual "benefit" of getting into the hospital sooner, these subjects said that the research benefited them psychologically.

I. Before the research started, how well did you feel you understood the potential benefits to yourself?

R. Well, I really feel that I am having a benefit, because, you know, with my strong Catholic background even though I don't go to church now, it has been drilled into me how terrible it is to have an abortion. So this being able to help somebody else does make everything seem a little bit better. It makes you feel . . . you know, it relieves your mind. You contributed. You don't have to feel that you've done a selfish thing because you've done something good for somebody else perhaps. (#106, white)

R. It made me feel good. I feel like I'm doing something positive instead of just killing my baby. At least I was helping science. This was a great consolation.

I. Did you think the research would be of any direct medical benefit to yourself?

R. Not direct medical benefit. The only benefit I would get would be in my own mind if I was satisfied. It didn't help me at all; I didn't get any medical benefit out of it. I wasn't thinking of my own benefit; I was thinking of the benefit to others and how I could do something. (#101, white)

It may be of interest that the principal investigator in the abortion-starvation study showed considerable understanding of this aspect of his subjects' participation. In the preliminary interview he mentioned his belief that many of his subjects were grateful for the opportunity to participate in something that may ultimately prolong the lives of other fetuses; he contended that there was real psychological improvement in some cases and he specifically mentioned Catholic women. He also noted the religious symbolism of the fast itself, that one may do penance by fasting in order to atone for sins—in this case, either the "sin" that resulted in the need for abortion or the "sin" of the abortion itself.

It should also be briefly mentioned that in neither of the two committed starvation-abortion subjects was this desire to do something "positive" the sole reason they mentioned for their participation. Both also stressed their desire to get into the hospital at the earliest possible moment, as did all other starvation subjects. It should also be pointed out that, as their investment in and understanding of the research increased, some of the benefiting subjects in the starvation-abortion study developed a commitment to the research.

CONCLUSION

Subjects participate in research for distinctly different reasons. The subject typology was based not only on subjects' expressed reasons for participating, but also on their awareness of the research. Our typology includes, (1) unaware subjects who tended to be uneducated, black, and clinic patients, (2) unwilling subjects who tended to be highly educated women who learned in the labor room that they were to receive an experimental drug and felt they had no option of refusing, (3) indifferent subjects who also learned of the research in the labor room and who apparently went along with it without really making a conscious decision, (4) benefiting subjects who agreed to participate because of real or imagined benefits and who tended to be private patients and relatively highly educated, and (5) committed subjects who participated because of their belief in the importance of research and their desire to be of assistance.

Incidentally, nothing in my research suggests that the benefits to self-esteem that accrued to committed subjects could not have been more widely distributed had there been greater efforts to emphasize the altruistic possibilities of the research in the recruitment of subjects. Many people clearly derive feelings of accomplishment and a sense of satisfaction from doing something of benefit to others. While such aspects of research could be overemphasized by researchers and create guilt among people who do not want to participate, the fact remains that the research situation is an excellent opportunity for researchers to educate members of the public. And it is true that a volunteer who is not aware of how his participation benefits medical knowledge and possibly other patients is deprived of something that might make his participation more meaningful. I return to this point in the last chapter.

NOTES

1. Renée C. Fox, *Experiment Perilous* (Glencoe: Free Press, 1959).
2. Renée C. Fox, "Some Social and Cultural Factors in American Society Conducive to Medical Research on Human Subjects," *Clinical Pharmacology and Therapeutics,* 4 (1960), 423–443. Stewart Perry in *The Human Nature of Science* (New York: Free Press, 1966) also emphasizes the deep concern for patients, which underlies researchers' "toughness defense" (pp. 65–66). In a more recent article written with Judith P. Swazey, Fox continues to speak of the "typically close" relations between most physician-investigators and their patient-subjects. Swazey and Fox, "The Clinical Moratorium: A Case Study of Mitral Valve Surgery," in *Experimentation with Human Subjects,* Paul A. Freund, ed. (New York: George Braziller, 1970), pp. 325–357.
3. John J. Lally and Bernard Barber, "'The Compassionate Physician': Frequency and Social Determinants of Physician-Investigator Concern for Human Subjects," *Social Forces,* 53 (December 1974). Only 17 percent of the nearly 400 investigators surveyed responded affirmatively to the question, "Have you *ever* found yourself becoming involved emotionally with the people serving as subjects in your research to an extent greater than you deem desirable for a researcher?"
4. Henry K. Beecher, *Research and the Individual: Human Studies* (Boston: Little, Brown, 1970), p. 24.
5. Henry K. Beecher, "Ethics and Clinical Research," *New England Journal of Medicine,* 274 (1966), 1354–1360.
6. M. H. Pappworth, *Human Guinea Pigs: Experimentation on Man* (Boston: Beacon, 1968).
7. See, for example, Julius A. Roth, "Staff and Client Control Strategies in Urban Hospital Emergency Services," *Urban Life and Culture,* 1 (April 1972), 45.
8. Talcott Parsons, *The Social System* (New York: Free Press, 1964 [1951]), pp. 433–465.
9. John W. Thibaut and Harold H. Kelley, *The Social Psychology of Groups* (New York: Wiley, 1959). Most relevant to this particular point is Chapter 7, "Power and Dependence."
10. There are no indications of any explicit threats to withdraw services if the patients did not accede to the doctor's desires in this instance. Such choices are apparently not unusual in some settings, however (see Roth, *op. cit.,* p. 47). An unpublished paper I wrote on the basis of emergency room observations at Yale-New Haven Hospital in 1968 contains similar descriptions of a threat to withdraw services as a way of gaining patient "cooperation."
11. Anna Freud, "The Doctor-Patient Relationship," in Jay Katz, *Experimentation with Human Beings* (New York: Russell Sage, 1972), p. 635.

12. T. F. Fox, "The Ethics of Clinical Trials," *Medicolegal Journal,* 28 (1960), 132–141. Cited in Henry K. Beecher, *Research and the Individual,* p. 52.

13. Daniel C. Martin et al., "Human Subjects in Clinical Research—A Report of Three Studies," *New England Journal of Medicine,* 279 (1968), 1426–1431.

14. Ibid., p. 1429.

CHAPTER SEVEN

OTHER REASONS FOR
PARTICIPATING

At its inception, this study's primary focus was on subjects' reasons for participating in research. Thus, subjects were questioned extensively about their motivations for participating and the factors they considered in deciding to take part. The subject typology discussed in Chapter Six was partly based on some of these data; the benefiting and committed types reflected subjects' most important reason for participating (either designated as such by subjects or because it was the first reason they mentioned). The indifferent category represented subjects who were not able to give reasons for participating other than why they were induced or the request of a doctor.

However, the discussion of the subject typology in Chapter Six did not convey all of the richness of subjects' responses to my many questions concerning reasons for participating. Subjects often mentioned several different reasons for participating and factors they considered in their decisions. These data allow us considerable additional insight into subjects' motivations, their definitions of the situation, and their perceptions of various important elements of the research situation.

In this chapter we examine *all* reasons given by subjects for participating. (No responses from unaware subjects are included, since I am concerned here with *stated* reasons for participation in the study.) Data from both free-response and fixed-alternative questions are presented, illustrated with quotations from interviews with subjects. Finally, the power or impact of the various decision factors on the ultimate decisions of subjects will be considered.

FREE-RESPONSE QUESTIONS

In both interviews, labor-induction subjects were asked free-response questions* about their reasons for volunteering to become research subjects.
Subjects' responses to these open-ended questions about their reasons for
participating and the factors they considered fell into several categories, as
shown in Table 15. The table presents subjects' responses at both the first
and the second interviews.

Perhaps the most striking thing about Table 15 is the larger number of
responses from labor-induction subjects in the second interviews as compared to first interviews. The aware subjects averaged almost three reasons
(2.96) for participation at the first interview, which took place in the labor
room shortly after the drug infusion began. At the second interview,
scheduled in the first few days after the induction procedure had been completed, subjects mentioned almost four reasons (3.86) apiece. The increase
was perhaps due to the fact that the first interview was done when subjects
had other things on their minds; it may have also resulted from the fact
that subjects had some time for reflection before the second interview.
Also, subjects were generally more talkative throughout the second interview. In few cases, however, did the second interview responses reflect a

**Table 15. Reasons for Participation: Responses to Free-
Response Questions (Aware Labor-Induction Subjects)**

Responses	First Interview ($N = 28$)	Second Interview ($N = 30$)
Wanted or needed to have labor induced	89%[a]	100%[a]
This was how the doctor wanted it done	64%	73%
Medical self-benefit from research	14%	27%
Convenience; being able to make plans	36%	53%
Benefit to others or to medical science	7%	17%
Safety; absence of risk	29%	47%
Recommended by own doctor	39%	43%
Other	18%	27%

[a] Subjects could and did give more than one reason for participation.

* These free-response questions were asked before any other items concerning reasons for participation so they would not elicit responses suggested by such other questions (see Appendix
B).

basic difference from the first interview responses as to reasons for agreeing to participate.*

Not all the responses given by subjects in answer to the question "Why did you decide (agree) to participate in the study?" really answered the question. The two most common responses in Table 15—reasons why the subject wanted or needed to be induced and the fact that a doctor asked her to do so—were not really answers to the question but were steps in the chain of events leading (supposedly) to a decision by the subject. Such answers reflect three problems in the consent process.

First, the large number of subjects who responded with the reason why they wanted or needed to be induced reflects, I believe, a confusion on the part of many subjects about what was or was not research.

Second (and this partially accounts for the first problem), most subjects did not have any conception of alternatives. Without the knowledge that there were alternative methods of being induced, the reasons why one wanted or needed to be induced would indeed be the reasons why one agreed to be in the research. And, in fact, most subjects were unable to tell me what alternative they had to being induced in the research, as was seen at the end of Chapter Five.

Third, in addition to reflecting a lack of awareness of alternatives, those who said they agreed because that is what the doctor wanted them to do illustrate a most difficult problem in reaching informed consent. Many subjects are anxious to please their physician and to comply with his wishes. Indeed, cooperation with a physician is part of the expectations of the sick role.[1] Many did not understand that being asked to consent to a research procedure entails a role obligation (the decision) that goes beyond the usual role obligations of patients. The phenomenon of acquiescence helps to explain why so many subjects, when asked why they agreed to participate, said it was because they had wanted or needed to be induced and this was how the physician proposed to do it.

The acquiescence phenomenon is not the only thing at work here, however. Approximately 60 percent (mostly private patients) of those who said they participated because their physician wanted them to further stated that their physician *recommended* it. This implies an awareness of options and that their physician's recommendation was one input into their decision-process. It is important to note, however, that talk of physicians' *recommendations* came from only 25 percent of *all* subjects in the labor-induction study. The rest, including the unaware subjects, apparently perceived their physician's wishes in stronger terms, that is, as a "doctor's

---

* In the few cases where a subject did shift her major reason for participation between the first and second interviews, the reason given in the first interview was used as the basis for categorizing a subject into the subject typology, as described earlier.

order." Or, because of the acquiescence phenomenon, they never stopped to consider the nature of what they were being presented with.

Like the "doctor's recommendation" responses, one other line in Table 15 reflects a factor considered in the decision rather than a positive reason why the decision was made. These were responses concerning risk or safety of the procedure. Most of these responses were of the "As long as it's not harmful, I'll go along with it" variety. I believe that subjects agreed more because it was "not unsafe" than because it was "safe." In the second interviews fewer than half the respondents (and fewer than 30 percent at the first interview) even mentioned risks or safety as a consideration, although this is clearly a relevant consideration in a drug investigation.

In summary, the most common free-responses in Table 15 reflect confusion among subjects about what elements of their inductions were "research," indicate a lack of awareness of alternatives or options to participation, and suggest widespread acquiescence rather than positive decision-making. Personal benefits were mentioned by large numbers of aware subjects, reflecting the earlier finding that 71 percent of the *aware* labor-induction subjects participated primarily because of real or imagined personal benefits (medical or convenience). A few subjects, all of whom were discussed in the section on committed subjects, mentioned benefit to others or to science as a reason for their participation; for only two was this the major reason. Fewer than half of the aware labor-induction subjects reported giving thought to the safety or risks of the research, and around 40 percent indicated that the recommendation of their own physician was a factor in their decisions.

Before leaving Table 15, let us turn briefly to the last line, "other" responses. Eighteen percent of subjects in the first interview and 27 percent in the second interview gave responses in addition to those already discussed. These additional reasons for participation were:

	Number of Subjects
Had no choice	2
Faith in the hospital and medical school	2
Curiosity	1
Financial considerations	1
In order to be induced before own doctor went on vacation	1
In order to be induced by particular member of ob/gyn group	1
Believed it would be less painful	1
Had "confidence in the doctors"	1
Received "logical explanations to my questions"	1

Some of these responses, such as the feeling of "no choice" reported by two unwilling subjects and faith in the institution or physicians, have already been discussed. The response concerning financial considerations came early in the interviewing period when a day's free hospitalization was being offered (an incentive that was dropped shortly thereafter); this subject, however, said this was not an important consideration for her. Two private patients used the study as a way of being with their own doctors, one of whom was going on vacation the next week; the other subject was going to have to be induced anyway in a few days, and the study gave her an opportunity to be induced by her favorite physician in her private ob/gyn group. The response concerning less pain, like some of the "medical benefit" responses cited earlier, was not based on fact. It was probably a projection of the subject's own wishes or was perhaps based on a confused notion of just what the research was—that is, the subject may have meant less pain compared to going into labor without induction. The woman who said that she went ahead because she received "logical explanations to her questions" was one of the unwilling subjects who would have preferred not to participate. She learned of the particulars of the research after admission, and asked so many questions that the research staff complained about her, even to me. But in the end, the staff was able to satisfy her enough that she went ahead with her induction in the study, albeit unhappily.

In my precoding scheme, I had anticipated two types of possible responses that were in fact not given by any of the subjects. No subject told me, in answer to free-response questioning, that she participated because her husband, other relatives, or friends thought that she should. Also, no subject told me that she participated because she felt that it might affect the care she would receive in the hospital. Both of these possible reasons did come up, however, in response to specific fixed-alternative questions, discussed in the next section.

Some of the consent difficulties raised in this section—subjects' confusion about what comprised the research study, the necessity of knowledge of options in a genuine decision-making process, and the problem of subject acquiescence and lack of awareness of the differing requirements of the subject and patient roles—are discussed in more detail in the next chapter on the vagaries of informed consent.

FIXED-ALTERNATIVE QUESTIONS

In addition to the free-response items, subjects were asked a series of structured, fixed-alternative questions about the reasons they participated and the factors they considered. These items included subjects' perception of 14 factors that I thought might be possible considerations in participation decisions. For each factor about which a subject showed awareness, she was asked how much thought she gave to the factor, and how important the factor was in her decision. Precoded response choices were read to subjects and ranged, respectively, from "no thought" and "not at all important" to "very much thought" and "very important."*

Table 16 presents the percentage of *aware* labor-induction subjects reporting perception of each of the 14 factors, and the percentage indicating that each factor was "somewhat" or "very important" in their decision to participate. The "how much thought" variables will not be presented, with three exceptions, because responses to them were so similar to responses to the "importance to the decision" variable that they contributed little additional information. However, for perception of risk, expectation of pain or discomfort, and fear of the unknown, the responses concerning "how much thought" was given to each factor are used rather than how important to the decision each factor was. This is because these factors were considerations that were *thought about* rather than being positive reasons why decisions were made.

Since each item taps a slightly different dimension, we should briefly examine each of the decision-factors contained in the fixed-alternative questions. Aspects already discussed in Chapter Six are touched on only lightly.

Direct Medical Benefit to Self.   When asked "At the time you decided to participate—did you think that the research (study) would be of any direct medical benefit to yourself?" 15 subjects said yes, 1 said maybe (combined with yes response in Table 16), and 13 said no. The benefits that subjects referred to were similar to those discussed in the section on benefiting subjects, although most benefiting subjects talked about convenience and ability to make plans, rather than medical benefit, as the reason for their participation. Here the question pertained to "medical benefits."

Subjects were asked to describe the benefits they had in mind. The benefit most commonly mentioned by subjects here was the nonexistent one of the new drug being either "quicker" or "easier." The research was intended, of course, to determine whether that was true. Five subjects gave this type of response. Some examples follow:

R.   If the research drug was used it would be quicker, I suppose. As far as a real benefit, I don't see that I had any real benefit from it. The personal benefit was to make it easier. (#03, white, private)

* An examination of the questionnaire (Appendix B, especially pp. 276–281) will clarify how this series of questions operated.

Table 16. Perception of Decision-Related Factors and Importance of the Factors to Participation Decisions (Aware Labor-Induction Subjects)

Factors	Percent Giving Positive Response	Percent Indicating Factor Is "Somewhat" or "Very" Important	(N)
Believed there was direct medical benefit to self	55%	48%	29
Believed there were risks of complications from research	27%	47%[a]	30
Expected pain or discomfort from research	17%	—	30
Believed inconvenience would result from research	3%	3%	30
Expressed belief that the research might produce knowledge that might help self or loved ones sometime in the future	60%	23%	30
Was afraid because did not know what to expect	30%	17%[a]	30
Believed that being in the research or refusing to participate might affect way treated in the hospital	7%	7%	30
Believed that it would be an interesting experience or was curious about what it would be like	73%	30%	30
Perceived that the researchers felt strongly that she should participate	24%	10%	29
Expected financial benefit	13%	—	30
Believed that it would help the researchers	87%	33%	30
Perceived strong family feelings either for or against participation	37%	17%	30
Believed that her participation might help to advance medical science	80%	27%	30
Felt that she knew at least "a little" about the researchers before participation began	40%	30%	30

[a] Indicates percentage of subjects giving "some thought" or "very much thought" to the factor.

H. She had the impression that this would be a way to finish faster than the other thing. Because with a new one, it should be better than the other ones, so that she would be out of there earlier. (Husband of #15, Puerto Rican, clinic)

R. I asked them if it were so different from the other drug they were using . . . if it were more effective than the other drug. They said it was proven to be. They said it would be more effective than the other one. So I was willing to give it a try. (#17, black, clinic)

It is not clear why these subjects believed that they were getting a better drug by taking part in the study, although the last subject said that she was so informed. The second quotation reflects the belief that "if it is new, it must be better." The research nurses commonly guessed at which medication a patient was receiving, and usually assumed the experimental drug was being used in cases in which labor began quickly or progressed rapidly. This indicated that they too believed that the experimental drug was better. Needless to say, such beliefs are a primary reason for the use of double-blind methodology in such studies.

Four subjects who gave positive responses to the question of medical benefit were unable to tell me what benefit they would receive from participating in the *study*; they simply stated their belief that labor-induction (not the research per se) would benefit them. For example:

R. It was benefiting me because it was getting things done. (#12, white, private)

R. It would help me with the baby. (#43, black, clinic)

Only 2 of the 30 aware subjects responded with benefits that subjects actually received through participation—that fetal monitoring equipment would be used and that their labor would be followed particularly closely because two full-time nurses were working on the project. In the words of one of these women:

R. They said they would monitor the baby's heart and that they would have someone with me at all times. I felt this was beneficial. Rather than just have someone pop in and out every hour or so. (#45, white, private)

Clearly then, most subjects had a poor understanding of the benefits of participation. But however poorly informed subjects were about the medical benefits accruing to them through participation in the labor-induction study, there were indications that personal benefit is a powerful factor in participation decisions. Twelve of the 14 subjects who believed that there was medical benefit (whether real or fancied) to themselves reported that this was an important factor in their decision to participate in the research.

Examination of the data on perception of medical benefit and the importance of medical benefit in the decision process showed no distinct differences by educational level or private-clinic status. With such small numbers, only striking differences of this sort would be worth mentioning.

Risks of Complications.   To the question, "Were there any risks of complications involved?" 8 subjects said yes, 20 said no, and 2 said they did not know. (This latter response referred to subjects' own lack of knowledge, not to the fact that there were unknown risks involved in using an experimental drug.) All 8 subjects who said there was a risk acknowledged, in varying degrees of explicitness and clarity, that there might be unknown risks. Their comments were presented earlier. Only one clearly indicated that she had been specifically informed on this point, however.

As seen earlier, those who believed there were no risks repeatedly told me that this is what they had been told; it is possible that they were told something like "we haven't had any problems with it" and translated that into their own belief that there was no risk. The consent form, it should be pointed out, *did* explicitly mention the factor of unknown risk by noting that "Although adverse effects are possible with any new drug, none have been noted with [the experimental drug]." Most subjects apparently noticed the latter rather than the former clause in that sentence, because 22 of 30 reporting said that they knew of no risks. (This is in addition, we should recall, to the 20 subjects who did not even know an experimental drug was being used.) The factors that account for these findings are examined in the next chapter, which is devoted to issues and problems in the consent process.

All aware subjects were asked how much thought they gave to the question of risks, whether or not they believed there were any. Several (7 of 16) of the subjects who said there were no risks reported giving "some" or "a great deal" of thought to the question of risk. Of those who acknowledged the possibility of risk or who did not know whether there were risks, 7 of 10 gave "some" or a "great deal" of thought to risks.

Awareness of and concern about risks in the labor-induction study was positively associated with subjects' educational level.* This is not

* Among the 8 subjects who recognized the possibility of unknown risks were 6 of the 13 aware subjects with at least some college, and 2 of the 11 high school graduates. None of the 6

surprising, since it is likely that well-educated subjects brought a greater general awareness of risks and experimentation to the situation, and may also have been more careful readers of the consent form. The difference also shows that any verbal efforts made by the researchers to inform subjects about risks were not successful with subjects who had less than some college education.

Pain or Discomfort. To the question, "Did you believe that there would be any pain or discomfort involved in the study?" 3 subjects said yes, 2 said maybe (combined with yes responses on Table 16), 24 said no, and 1 did not know. Once again, subjects apparently confused the research aspects of the study with what would have been done had research not been taking place; only one subject clearly did have research procedures in mind:

R.   I thought about [pain or discomfort] because I knew that they would
be putting the electrodes on the baby's head. But I'm not one to worry
about pain. I guess I have a high pain tolerance or something. (#03,
white, private)

For whatever reason, however, not a single subject said that the anticipation of pain or discomfort was an important consideration in her decision. Perhaps this is because they assumed that whatever discomfort might be involved would be only a marginal increment to what would be necessitated by labor and birth, no matter how it was done.

Those subjects who anticipated pain or discomfort were not distinctive in any way by education, private-clinic status, or race. All categories on these three variables were found among the five subjects who perceived the possibility of pain or discomfort in the study.

Inconvenience. To the question, "Did you believe that the study would mean any inconvenience to you?" only one subject replied in the affirmative.* She had in mind the fetal monitoring procedures and noted that

---

* Actually, the item on inconvenience would have been more useful as an affirmative question, that is, "Did you believe that the study would mean any *convenience* to you?" As pointed out earlier, the largest category of subjects were those who participated for their own benefit, and the benefit mentioned by the majority of these had to do with convenience and the ability to make plans because delivery would be scheduled. Without such an item in the questionnaire, the factor of convenience cannot be compared with the other factors covered in the fixed-alternative questions.

---

aware subjects with less than a high school education recognized the possibility. Among those who gave "some" or "very much" thought to the question of risks (whether or not they believed risks were present) were 9 of 13 subjects with at least some college, 3 of the 12 with high school degrees, and 1 of 6 with less education.

"the things they wouldn't ordinarily do will be better, but they won't be pleasant" (02, white, clinic). This subject, incidentally, was a registered nurse, and she reported giving "a great deal of thought" to this aspect of the situation.

Produce Knowledge That Might Help Self or Loved Ones in Future.   To the question, "Did you believe that the research might produce knowledge that might help you or your loved ones sometime in the future?" 18 subjects said yes, 10 said no, and 2 did not know. Only 7 of these women said that this was a somewhat or very important factor in their decisions to participate.

Subjects with high school education were slightly more likely to respond to this aspect than were subjects with more or less education, although the differences and numbers are too small to allow us to speak with confidence.* If the small difference is real, it is consistent with an hypothesis offered later in this chapter, that subjects with intermediate amounts of education are more likely than subjects with either more or less education to glamorize research.

Fear of Not Knowing What to Expect.   To the question, "Were you at all afraid because you did not know what to expect?" 10 aware labor-induction subjects said yes and 20 said no. Of those saying yes, 5 reported being "a little bit" afraid, 1 was "somewhat" afraid, and 4 were "very much" afraid. A total of 6 subjects reported that they gave at least "some" thought to their fear of not knowing what was going to happen; this included the 4 who reported that they were "very much" afraid and 2 who were "a little bit" afraid.

Highly educated subjects may be slightly underrepresented among those who reported being fearful and for whom this was given more than "very little" thought. However, the small differences and few cases make it impossible to discuss this with any confidence.†

---

* Among the 18 who answered affirmatively to the original question were 7 of 13 aware subjects with at least some college, 9 of 11 subjects with high school diplomas, and 2 of the 6 subjects with less than high school. Among the 7 who reported that this belief was an important factor in their decision were 2 of the 13 subjects with at least some college, 5 of the 12 with high school diplomas, and none of the 6 subjects with less education.

† Among the 10 who reported fear were 3 of the 13 aware subjects with college experience, 4 of the 11 with high school diplomas, and 3 of the 6 with less education. Among the 5 reporting giving "some" or "very much" thought to their fears were 1 of the 13 subjects with college experience (and she had not completed college), 2 of the 11 subjects with high school degrees, and 2 of the 6 subjects with less education.

Affect the Care One Would Receive. Two subjects responded to the question, "Did you believe that being in this research (or refusing to participate) might affect the care you would receive or the way you were treated while in the hospital?" by indicating that they believed that their refusal to participate would have had negative consequences.

I. In what way did you believe it would affect you?

R. In a negative way if I refused.

I. How?

R. Well . . . um . . .

I. That you might be sent home or another way?

R. Either that or they might be annoyed because we didn't do it and therefore, in some way, not give me the attention I would require. (#45, white, private)

R. If I *didn't* use it [the new drug] it would affect the relationship, rather than if I *did* use it. (#24, white, private)

Both of these cases were discussed in some detail in the earlier section on unwilling subjects; here we only need to point out that concern that the quality of care one receives may be threatened by a refusal to participate in research is completely alien to the concept of *consent*. There is *no* evidence that the researchers tried to put such pressure on subjects, or that these subjects felt such pressure from the researchers, however. Both of these subjects believed that refusal would jeopardize their relationship with their private physician, as was discussed earlier. Incidentally, they did not have the same private physician.

Although there is no evidence that any physician intended to apply the kind of pressure to participate that was perceived by these subjects, the pressure was very real as a perception. This suggests that conscious efforts should be made to be sure a prospective subject understands that his participation is voluntary, that he has options, and that his care is in no way an issue. If these things are not made explicit, some subjects will not recognize their own responsibility in decision-making, and other subjects may feel that pressure is being applied for participation.

As seen earlier, some subjects did recognize the positive benefits with respect to extra care and special monitoring that came with being in the research. These benefits were also mentioned in response to this question. For example:

R. I thought accepting it would probably entail better care. But that refusing wouldn't have affected it one way or the other.

I. You mean the routine procedures of the research would be beneficial. The monitoring?

R. Yes, and the follow-up on the baby would be even better care. But there would be no hard feelings if . . . [I refused to participate]. (#34, white, private)

R. Just that being in the study, I felt that for the actual birth I might get extra care. But not for the duration of it.

I. But you didn't feel that there would be recriminations if you refused?

R. Oh, no. (#46, white, private)

Curiosity. To the question, "Did you believe that it would be an interesting experience? That is, were you curious what it would be like?" most aware labor-induction subjects (22 of 30) said yes. Three said they were "a little bit curious or interested," while 16 were "somewhat" and 12 were "very" curious or interested. In comparing the 11 subjects who expressed little or no curiosity or interest with the 18 who were somewhat or very interested or curious, subjects with intermediate levels of education again seem to be the most fascinated with the idea of medical research, although again the numbers and differences are too small to allow for much confidence.*

Nine subjects reported that their interest in or curiosity about the research was a "somewhat" or "very important" factor in their decision to participate in the research. Little difference by education was apparent.

Perhaps a note of explanation should be added concerning why some subjects did not believe that participation in a research project would be interesting, or why any person would not be curious to know what such an experience would be like. Two different explanations were offered by the subjects themselves.

* Among the 18 subjects who were at least "somewhat" interested in or curious about the research were 6 of the 13 subjects with at least some college, 9 of the 11 subjects with high school diplomas, and 3 of the 6 subjects with less education.

I. Were you curious what it would be like?

R. Not really. I really didn't think about it that much. And I didn't realize what they were going to be doing to the *extent* of what they were going to be doing. I thought they were just going to be watching, really, an inducement. I did not realize that this was a whole separate thing. (#34, white, private)

This subject is suggesting that she was not more interested or curious about the research because she did not understand what was involved. Thus, the widespread lack of understanding among the subjects in this study may have acted to deprive subjects of an experience that could have been interesting or even exciting had they understood it better.

The second reason offered by a subject is as follows:

R. No, [I wasn't curious what it would be like]. [laughed] Someone who had never had a baby before might think it was going to be different under an experiment, but having had a baby before—labor is labor whether . . . (#32, white, private)

Researchers Felt Strongly. To the question, "Did the doctor(s) doing the research feel strongly that you should participate?" 7 aware labor-induction subjects said yes, 3 said no, and 19 said they did not know how the researchers felt. Since the "don't know" response indicated an absence of pressure, this response was combined with those saying no in Table 16. The larger number of such answers, however, may be important in and of itself as an indicator of lack of contact between the researchers and subjects before the decision was made to participate, or at least a lack of any explicit understanding between researcher and subject that the participation decision was in the subject's hands. Such reasons were suggested by subjects' comments:

I. Did the doctors doing the research feel strongly that you should participate?

R. Well, he . . . Dr. C [the co-investigator] didn't pressure me or anything. I mean, he just came in and explained and everything. Took it more as a matter of course. I had signed [the consent form] already. So I don't feel as though he . . . you know. (#45, white, private)

R. I don't know whether they did [feel strongly] or not, but they just seemed like they thought it was best for me to participate in it. (#25, black, clinic)

R. They didn't say either way because I didn't talk to a doctor about research. (#28, black, clinic)

Three subjects, however, responded to the question with an explicit statement that the doctor had not made his feelings known because it was the subject's decision to make:

R. No, he didn't harp on it or emphasize on it. He said it would be good. (#04, white, private)

R. It was really up to me. If I wanted to I could; if I didn't want to that was OK. (#23, white, clinic)

R. I don't think they did [have strong feelings]. I don't think they felt strongly one way or the other. It was appreciated, I imagine, but of no really terribly great importance. (#30, white, clinic)

The last statement was from one of the two committed subjects in the labor-induction study.

Four subjects (including the last one quoted) indicated that they felt the researchers felt a strong need for subjects and were glad to get them:

R. Strongly? Actually they were glad to have me participate, but if I had said no I doubt if they were going to hate me. But I think they were kind of glad to have me because they haven't had that many. Like they were saying that they wouldn't have another until next week. (#12, white, private)

R. I think they were glad to find someone. [laughed] I heard one of them say they have a hard time finding people. That made me feel like they might take people off the street, like those body snatchers. [laughed] (#19, white, private)

None of these subjects, however, expressed any feeling that the researchers had pressured them into participating.

Two subjects felt that the researchers would not have asked them to participate if they had not felt strongly that the woman should participate. Rather than talking about pressure from the researchers, however, both of these women exhibited confusion (mentioned earlier and discussed at length in the next chapter) concerning the role of research subject:

I. Did the doctors doing the research feel strongly that you should participate?

R. Since I was a valuable subject, I would think so, yes . . . I knew they thought I should. Otherwise they would never have taken me down there in the first place. So after having them explain it to me, I thought about it some.

I. How important was this as a factor in your decision?

R. Not very important, because they didn't actually pressure me about it. (#17, black, clinic)

The role confusion I referred to is exhibited in the subject's belief that she would not have been asked to participate if the researchers had not thought she "should." She does not seem to recognize that researchers might have other reasons for asking a person to become a research subject. The second woman who showed the same role confusion said:

R. They wouldn't have gone ahead and given me the stuff if they didn't think I was going to deliver.

I. How important was this as a factor in your decision?

R. He did check me before he hooked me up. They put me on a scale as to how good my chances were of delivering. If he had said that I was low on the scale, I don't think I would have done it. (#04, white, private)

The latter statement was completely erroneous. I was told by the principal investigator that this subject had not been very suitable because she was not as "ripe" as he would prefer. He was not pleased with her inclusion, but the decision had essentially been made by her private obstetrician. If she had been his own patient, the principal investigator said that he would not have induced her.

This illustrates an aspect of the research situation that cannot be thoroughly investigated within the confines of the present study—the extent to which an investigator, depending on other physicians for subjects and having to deal with these physicians on a continuing basis, may have to do things he may regard as unsound medical practice. At least two other examples of similar situations came to my attention. One involved another subject whom the researchers did not think should be induced (at least the indications for induction were marginal), but who had been preselected for them by a private physician. The other case involved a private patient whose induction the researchers were prepared to call a failure; she was not going to deliver. Her private physician, however, made the decision to rupture her membranes, and she went ahead and delivered. The principal investigator believed that this particular rupture of membranes could have never been justified in terms of the research, and that as a researcher he would not have done it. However, the private physician who did not have to examine his motives—he did not have research considerations pushing him to act in certain ways—was able to make this decision and carry it through.

We should also add that, with the few cases available, there was no apparent relationship between subjects' perceptions of researchers' feelings that they should participate and subjects' educational level or clinic-private status.

Finally, only three subjects, with no apparent common characteristics, reported that their perception of the researchers' feelings was a "somewhat" or "very" important factor in their decision to participate.

Financial Benefit.   Four subjects in the labor-induction study responded affirmatively to the question, "Did you believe that there would be any financial benefit or special accommodations if you participated?" These were the first four subjects I interviewed, and all referred to one day's free hospitalization, a benefit that was dropped thereafter. In fact, it was dropped in the middle of the fourth subject's involvement; she was told by her private physician a few days before admission that she would get a free day, but was not told that this policy ended at the end of the month. She was admitted on the first day of the next month, and was upset about this, feeling that she had been misled.

The principal investigator said in the preliminary interview that he was concerned that his offer of a free day would be too strong an inducement for participation; he did not want people to volunteer because of such considerations. Rather, he saw the free day as a reward. Therefore, he said that subjects were not to be told of the free day until after they had agreed to participate. I learned nothing directly about how this policy worked in practice, but, for whatever reason, none of the subjects said it was of more than "very little importance" in their decision to participate. Only one subject reported giving as much as "some" thought to the financial aspect of the research. The financial aspect, then, was not a powerful motivating factor in that particular situation.

Likewise in the starvation-abortion study. The few subjects who understood how their participation in the starvation study could save them money nevertheless indicated that this was not an important consideration to them or an important reason why they agreed to participate.

There are several possible reasons why financial benefits were not an important factor among these subjects—the way these benefits were presented to subjects, or because there were other, more important factors to be considered, or because the financial inducements were not sufficiently large. The finding does suggest, however, that it is possible to attach a financial reward to participation in research without that reward assuming undue importance as a motivating factor.

Help the Researchers.   To the question, "Did you believe that it would help the researchers if you participated?" 28 of 30 responding subjects said yes. Of the two saying no, one said that she had not thought about it, and the other interpreted the question somewhat differently, as she responded "It would help them no more than any other woman."

The overwhelming response, though, was that subjects believed it would help the researchers. Subjects were asked in what way it would be of help. I was particularly interested in whether subjects perceived that researchers have career interests that are advanced through successful research. Not one subject mentioned this at this particular point, however. Twenty-four subjects said that their participation would help the researchers learn more and thus medicine would advance, and the other two who responded said it would help the doctors know better how to treat future patients. Thus, even though asked what might seem to be a leading question about how their participation would help the researchers, no subjects showed awareness of the career aspect. This is additional evidence that subjects were not very aware of the key differences between physician as therapist and physician as researcher. Hence, they were not aware of the differing role requirements of patient and subject, with implications to be discussed in the next chapter.

Although almost all aware labor-induction subjects acknowledged that their participation would help the researchers, only one-third indicated that this was either a "somewhat" or a "very important" reason for their participation.* Those who had the highest level of education were least likely to indicate that helping the researchers was an important reason for their participation. This may have something to do with the way they were selected rather than their basic interest in research or desire to help others. It should be recalled that those with high education were most likely to have a private physician. Private physicians, we argued in Chapter Four, were much more likely than house staff physicians to involve their patients in the research for reasons that the patients knew about. Such reasons usually involved meeting the patients' self–defined needs—medical or convenience. Therefore, patients with high education were most likely to have

---

* Among these 10 subjects were 2 of the 12 responding subjects with at least some college experience, 5 of 11 with high school diplomas, and 3 of the 6 with less education.

known of personal benefits from participation at the time they made their decisions; furthermore, they were most likely to have made a decision regarding participation before they came into the hospital and before they ever met the researchers. Thus, their decisions were unlikely to have involved their perception of the researchers' needs.

Family Feelings Regarding Participation. To the question, "Did any of your family feel strongly one way or the other about your participation?" 11 aware labor-induction subjects said yes, 13 said no, and 7 indicated that they had no opportunity to discuss it with their families. Not all of those who said their families had no strong feelings actually discussed it with any family members, but they were judged to have had an opportunity to do so if they had so desired. Those who had such opportunity were those who had been unaccompanied to the labor room and who learned of the research for the first time there; many such women, of course, ended up as unaware subjects and are not included in this discussion.

Of the women reporting strong family feelings, five said that family members favored participation, one said she received mixed opinions, and five reported family opposition to participation. No educational differences between these groups were apparent.

Five women reported that feelings of family members were a "somewhat" or "very important" factor in their decisions; five said that they were of "very little" or no importance. Four of the five who received positive opinions from family said that family opinions were important to their decision; four of the five who received split or negative opinions said that family feelings were not important. One possible interpretation of this is consistent with the fact that, for several reasons, subjects were generally in a position that made it difficult to refuse to participate. Furthermore, all were anxious to have their babies, and the research presented them with the earliest opportunity to do just that. It is not surprising, then, that women took seriously family members who felt that participation was a good idea, and tended to ignore those who advised against it. One subject said that she responded to her husband's negative opinion by telling him that "it had to be done," and said that his opinion was "not a factor" in her decision (#16, white, clinic).

There are indications that some of the advice received did not deal with the research itself, but was directed at the idea of induction, as in the following response:

R. Some did [feel strongly]. Some thought . . . well, a lot of them felt like when it's time for the baby to come it will come.

I.   And they felt you shouldn't do it?

R.   Yes. (#43, black, clinic)

This exhibits the same confusion between research and nonresearch aspects of the procedure that has already been mentioned.

A final note on seeking advice from husband and relatives: two subjects who found out about the research for the first time in the labor room (and who therefore were already committed to going ahead) said that they felt incapable of making a decision at that point. They turned to their husbands for a decision, even though they reported that they usually made this type of a decision themselves. One of them suggested a possible reason for this behavior, which they regarded as unusual in themselves:

R.   I didn't say [to my husband] "the decision is up to you," but I said "Well, what should we do" and I really passed the buck to him. Which is awful, because if something happened, then I could blame him. Human nature. [laughed] (#45, white, private)

Overall, it is hard to measure the potential impact of family feelings on the decision process from this study, because the opportunities for such involvement, as well as the amount of time subjects had to consider the decision, varied so widely. The procedures that were followed with respect to informing subjects about the research clearly and effectively kept the family out of the decision-process for many subjects, and allowed them only a minor role with other subjects.

Help Advance Medical Science.   To the question, "Did you believe that your participation might help advance medical science?" 21 aware labor-induction subjects said yes, 3 said maybe (included with positive response in Table 16), and 6 said no. Of those saying no, the comments of several highly educated subjects indicated that they meant that they did not think about this aspect, not that they believed that the statement was untrue:

R.   I think I was too concerned about myself to start thinking about what it would do for others. (#24, white, private)

R.   I believe it now, but at the time I didn't give any thought to it. (#32, white, private)

A subject who said she was "not sure" indicated another sense in which subjects might fail to respond positively to the question:

R. Not really, no. I figured, you know, it was helping them, but it wasn't going to advance them very much.

I. You mean because you were just one person?

R. Yes. (#48, white, faculty patient)

But most subjects affirmed the belief that their participation would help advance medical science. Only 8 subjects, however, indicated that this was an important factor in their decision to participate. Among them were 2 of the 13 aware subjects with at least some college (neither of whom said it was a "very important factor"), 4 of the 11 subjects with high school diplomas (all of whom said it *was* a "very important factor"), and 2 of the 6 subjects with less education. These numbers, though very small, are consistent with the pattern of highly educated subjects being less likely to place a halo around "medical research."

Knowledge About the Researchers. To the final question in this series, "What did you know or how much did you know about the doctor(s) doing the research before the research started?" 1 subject said "a great deal," 6 said they had "some" knowledge of the researchers, 5 said they had "a little" knowledge, and 18 said they had no prior knowledge about the researchers.

Knowledge about the researchers came from several sources. Four subjects reported having had prior professional contacts with the principal investigator. Three other subjects' knowledge of the investigators was based on what they had been told by their own physician:

R. I knew that Dr. D respected Dr. P. I was very much dependent upon Dr. D's advice and feeling about this. He said that if some young guy that he knew nothing about was doing this, I wouldn't have gone into it. (#49, white, private)

R. Dr. D assured me that he was one of the very best. (#04, white, private)

R. Dr. D's word is OK by me. I have been going to him for 10 years. (#03, white, private)

Still another patient said that her knowledge of Dr. D's relationship with Dr. P was important:

R. I knew Dr. P, not from having met him, but from knowing that he takes care of Dr. D's patients, and also he is taking care of a friend of mine. I knew what he was doing, you know, as far as the word of mouth things that go around. (#22, white, private)

With the exception of the one faculty patient, all of the subjects who reported having at least "some" knowledge about the investigators were patients of the private obstetrician for whom the investigators covered when he was away.

Knowledge about the researchers was a powerful factor, because *every* patient who said she had at least "some" knowledge about the researchers reported that this was a "somewhat" or "very important" factor in the decision to participate. Overall, nine subjects indicated that knowledge about the researcher was a factor of this importance.

Three clinic patients indicated they had knowledge of the investigators. One did not give the source of her knowledge; one said that the knowledge that they were affiliated with that particular medical school and hospital was a "very important" factor in her decision; the third, a nurse, reported that she had read an article by the principal investigator and that this was a "somewhat" important factor in her decision because it showed that "they knew what they were doing, I figure." (#02, white, clinic)

Subjects' responses regarding knowledge of the investigators suggest two things. First, such knowledge can have great importance in reducing anxieties about the unknown elements involved in any research. Several of these women mentioned this. The patients of one obstetrician (Dr. D) seemed to be at a distinct advantage regarding peace of mind about the whole thing. Second, these responses also point up the obvious danger (not manifested in the present study) that patients can put so much faith in a physician as not to evaluate for themselves the factors involved in a research project. These dangers are heightened, of course, in situations where a physician is doing research on subjects with whom he has had past involvement, or for whom he is presently acting as physician-therapist as well as physician-investigator.

POWER OF DECISION FACTORS

A crude but potentially useful index of the power of the various decision factors can be constructed by examining the proportion of subjects perceiving the existence of a factor who indicated that the factor was an important one in their decision. Thus, for example, 12 of 14 subjects who perceived personal benefit from participation indicated that this was either "somewhat" or "very important" in their decision, an index score of .86. Table 17 lists the 14 factors about which subjects were asked in order of their power in decision processes. Since some factors involve very few cases and must be interpreted in that light, the numbers are also shown in the table.

The power of any particular factor will vary from study to study. Although the index scores in Table 17 are based on a single study involving relatively few cases, it is useful to point out certain things in Table 17, to speculate a bit on what accounts for the relative power of the factors in the present study, and to hypothesize about how this might differ in other types of medical research.

Risk, as seems appropriate in an investigatory drug study involving essentially normal subjects, was the most powerful factor, as measured here. Risk of complications was the only factor for which the number of subjects who perceived the factor to exist (that is, perceived that risks were present) was fewer than the number of subjects who reported giving much thought to the factor. In other words, several subjects who said no risks were present also reported giving thought to the question of risks. (For most items this was a logical impossibility, since it generally made little sense to ask a subject how much thought was given to something he reported not perceiving.) It must be remembered also that risk was a topic about which a high proportion of subjects were judged to be poorly informed. I would hypothesize that risk would rank high as a powerful decision factor in most research, except that which appears to be innocuous.

The second factor, perception that refusal to participate might affect the care one receives or the way one is treated, involved only two subjects. Nevertheless, I would hypothesize that the perception of pressure or a threat (real or imagined) would always be a powerful decision factor, whenever perceived, though probably at its highest in situations where the potential subject is in a dependent position, as these subjects certainly were. The power of this factor is further indicated by the fact that it was, or was closely related to, the primary reason for both of these subjects' participation. They were both unwilling subjects.

One subject mentioned inconvenience; it is difficult to speculate on the general power of this factor, but it may be hypothesized to vary inversely to perceived medical benefit in research and inversely to perceived risk as well. Probably where either risk or benefit is an important factor, inconvenience will recede in importance.

Medical benefit, not surprisingly in view of the large number of benefiting subjects in the labor-induction study, ranks high in power as a decision factor, even though most subjects had erroneous beliefs concerning the benefits they might receive. One would expect that the power of

Table 17. Power of Decision Factors (Labor-Induction Study)

Decision Factor	Number Perceiving Factor[a] (A)	Number Indicating Factor Important[b] (B)	Power Index (B/A) (C)
1. Risks of complications	8	14	1.75[c]
2. Participation or refusal might affect care	2	2	1.00
3. Inconvenience would result	1	1	1.00
4. Medical benefit to self would result	14	12	.86
5. Possessed knowledge about the researcher(s)	12	9	.75
6. Fear of not knowing what to expect	10	5	.50
6. Family had strong feelings	10	5	.50
8. Researchers had strong feelings	7	3	.43
9. Interesting experience; curiosity	22	9	.41
10. Knowledge might be produced that would help self or loved ones in future	18	7	.39
11. Participation would help the researchers	28	10	.36
12. Participation might help advance medical science	24	8	.33
13. Pain or discomfort might result	5	0	.00
14. Financial benefit	4	0	.00

[a] Responses are included only if subject responded to items making up both columns.

[b] Factor considered important if subject indicates the factor was "somewhat" or "very" important to decision, except factors 1, 3, 6 (fear), and 13. For these factors, subjects were asked only how much thought they gave to the factor; factor is considered important if subject indicated "some" or "very much" thought given to factor.

[c] Index scores of larger than unity were possible on factors (such as risk and pain) that could be important by their absence. Thus, the number of women who reported giving "some" or "very much" thought to the question of risks was larger than the number who reported believing that some risks were actually involved.

medical benefit as a decision variable would be closely related to the actual benefit present in a research project. At least where medical benefit is present one can expect it to be a decision factor, since presumably few researchers will fail to apprise a prospective subject of the benefit accruing from taking part in his research project (although they might not emphasize the aspects that would be most salient to patients). The variation in power of benefit as a factor might be muffled by two factors. First, there may be a tendency among researchers to inflate the benefits to subjects in their projects. Second, subjects (except for completely normal volunteers) may have a general tendency to overestimate the personal benefit to themselves when a physician asks them to take part in something, because many people apparently cannot conceive of a physician in a nontherapeutic role. That seems to be the case in the present study.

Knowledge about the researchers was a powerful factor in this study, and there is no reason to believe that this would not generally be the case. The same might be said about fear and the perception of strong family feelings. Whenever these factors are present they will probably show considerable power.

The power of perception of strong feelings on the part of the researchers can be hypothesized to vary with the actual extent to which the researcher makes active attempts to persuade. In the present study, little attempt was apparently made, and this was a relatively unimportant factor. The investigators, by confining their role to offering explanations in response to questions and by conducting themselves as if everything were routine (which it was to them), did little to draw a subject's attention to their feelings about the her participating. It is difficult to speculate on what might be the impact of a researcher's conducting himself in such a way that subjects perceive strong feelings on his part. Subjects who cannot separate the physician-researcher from the physician-therapist might be expected to respond positively; those who understand the essential difference between these two roles might be frightened off by such an approach.

Curiosity about the study or the belief that participation might be an interesting experience was relatively unimportant as a factor in this study, probably because subjects had more important things on their minds. They were, after all, about to give birth. Curiosity might be hypothesized to be of greatest power in studies where both risks and benefits are at a minimum, and in innocuous studies involving normal volunteers.

The three "altruistic" factors—belief that future knowledge might result, belief that the researchers would be helped, and belief that medical science might be advanced—all show relatively little power in the present labor-induction study. The same speculations as were made about curiosity and interest might apply, with the exception that where risk is high relative to benefit, we can hypothesize that altruistic factors would show more power, at least in the absence of coercion or ignorance of risk. The altruistic possibilities of volunteering probably must be made explicit by researchers before the factor will show much power.

Pain and discomfort showed no power in this study, probably because the subjects expected only a small increment in the considerable amount of pain and discomfort they expected to experience in any case. There is no reason to expect that the perception of expected pain and discomfort would generally be a factor of low power; it may be hypothesized to increase with the perception of greater increments of pain and discomfort resulting from a research project relative to the pain or discomfort already present.

Financial benefit also showed no power in this study. It would seem more likely to do so where medical benefits are low, risks are high, and financial benefits are high. In the present study, the relatively small financial benefits offered to the first few subjects were minor compared to other factors.

One factor of great power was not covered in the fixed-alternative questions upon which this discussion has been based. This is the factor of convenience (as opposed to inconvenience which *was* asked about) resulting from participation in the study. Convenience was a major consideration among subjects in *both* projects studied. If the proper questions had been asked, I believe that convenience would have had a high power index score, since most subjects did perceive that the research was their first chance to get admitted to the hospital, and the largest number gave this as their primary reason for volunteering.

Perception of alternatives or options to participation in research is another highly important variable that was not covered in the fixed-alternative questions. This important aspect would be difficult to assess by asking for subjects' ratings, however, since it is a factor of which many subjects may not be aware. Even if they participated because they knew of no alternatives, they might not themselves view this as the reason. Rather they might cite the need for the procedure, or the fact that the physician seemed to think that they should participate, as was done by numerous subjects in the labor-induction study. My own assessment is that most subjects in the labor-induction study had little conception of options (see Chapter Five) and this was a major reason for their participation.

Finally, it may be appropriate to note the potential utility of examining the power of decision factors in a study as an indicator of the quality of informed consent among its subjects. That is, one would expect subjects in a risky study to report considering risk. If a study has no benefit to subjects, measures of altruism should show considerable power. The point is that reasons offered by subjects for their participation can be useful evidence of the validity of the consent process in the study.

NOTE

1. Talcott Parsons, *The Social System* (New York: Free Press, 1964 [1951]), p. 437.

CHAPTER EIGHT

THE VAGARIES OF CONSENT

Our detailed discussion of the reasons why subjects volunteer and the factors they consider leads us again to the issue of informed consent. In earlier chapters it was shown that the participation of many subjects in the labor-induction study was not based on informed consent. There is no question but that informed consent was required in that study; the situation was covered unambiguously by PHS policy, the institution's peer review committee judged informed consent to be necessary, and the principal investigator acknowledged the need for it and used consent forms. Even so, problems of informed consent emerge as a central focus of this study, although it did not originate as a study of such problems.

In this chapter I want to present in a more systematic fashion the factors that can interfere with informed consent, using examples from the research projects I studied. Factors that have already been described at length will be only briefly mentioned here.

THE IMPORTANCE OF CONSENT

Informed consent, as Henry Beecher has put it, is the "central issue on which hang most of the ethical problems of human experimentation."[1] The findings of this study confirm that judgment. The meaning of "informed consent" was discussed in some detail at the beginning of Chapter Four, but that discussion was largely confined to the legal basis for the requirement of consent. Legal considerations give only a partial indication of the importance and functions of informed consent, however. Jay Katz sees informed consent as serving four main functions, and these provide a larger context against which to consider the need for informed consent.

Most clearly, requiring informed consent serves society's desire to respect each individual's autonomy and his right to make choices concerning his own life. Second, providing a subject with information about an experiment and encouraging him to be an active partner in the process may also increase the rationality of the experimentation process.

Third, securing informed consent protects the experimentation process by encouraging the investigator to question the value of the proposed project and the adequacy of the measures he has taken to protect subjects, by reducing civil and criminal liability for non-negligent injury to the subjects and by diminishing adverse public reaction to an experiment. Finally, informed consent may serve the function of increasing society's awareness about human research. For instance, the need to obtain consent from large numbers of potential donors for removal of their kidneys after death has led to an extensive program of information about renal transplantation. While the motivation for the information campaign was to recruit individual donors, it also enlightens the public at large.[2]

In his massive and extremely useful compendium of materials relating to human experimentation, Katz has devoted a section to each of these functions of consent.[3]

A NOTE ON INTERPRETATION OF MATERIALS IN THIS CHAPTER

Before we look at the problems that account for shortcomings in informed consent, we should point out that while researchers are responsible for seeing that informed consent takes place, there is no evidence that the researchers in the two projects studied *intended* that there be inadequacies in the consent process. These researchers did not dispute the ethical validity of the principle of informed consent as it applied to their research, and they apparently believed that the conduct of their research was satisfactory in this regard. Their willingness to cooperate with my interviews of their subjects is evidence of their good intentions. Their performance also shows evidence of this. Both projects (and the consent forms used) had the approval of the Clinical Research Committee, and, in the labor-induction study, consent forms were signed by each subject before the drug infusion began. In the starvation-abortion study, the actual signing of the consent form was more casual. It was always done sometime before the subject was discharged, but usually only after the fast had actually begun, sometimes 2 or 3 days into the fast. Nevertheless, informed consent was more the norm in that project, for reasons we mention later.

The point that the researchers followed the standard procedures in good faith is an important one,* because it suggests that the consent failures resulted from factors such as the way subjects became involved and the nature of medical research in a research-oriented medical school and hospital, rather than from idiosyncracies or intent of the investigators themselves. The factors to be discussed all undoubtedly occur in other studies at other times and places; there is no reason to believe that any of these factors is peculiar to these investigators or to the institution in which my study was done.

TYPES OF CONSENT PROBLEMS TO BE DISCUSSED

The concept of informed consent obviously contains two elements. There must be a *free decision* that is *based upon adequate information*. From these elements follow two general types of reasons by which the consent process can fail. Pressures and constraints can prevent free choice, or subjects can lack the information necessary to an informed decision. The distinction is not perfect; lack of information can inhibit one's freedom to refuse. But it does provide a convenient way for organizing the inadequacies in the consent process that can be identified in these two studies.

A third, more general reason for the widespread failure of informed consent is also discussed, although it was not a result of the specific procedures followed in the projects studied. It became apparent that many people have a poor understanding of the peculiar characteristics of the researcher—subject role relationship that distinguish it from the usual doctor-patient relationship, and that this lack of understanding interferes with the freedom of potential subjects to refuse to participate.

Problems with Free Decisions. The concept of consent implies the freedom to refuse. If a prospective subject does not feel that he has been presented with a choice, then it would seem to be impossible for a genuine consent process to take place.†

---

* This is in no way intended to suggest that conscious evasion of procedural requirements intended to protect subjects does not take place (see Chapter Three), but only that such evasion does not explain the consent shortcomings with which we are concerned here.

† A subject's freedom to refuse can be limited by factors over which the investigator has no control. For example, the individual who is dying of an incurable disease may have only limited freedom to refuse an experimental program that offers hope, however slight. To say that consent is not possible in such situations, however, would serve no purpose. The free decision-inhibiting factors discussed in this section are those over which the investigator has some degree of control.

> Valid consent is a contract between equals as far as it involves
> freedom to accept or reject. The investigator, with his superior
> knowledge, must overcome any tendency to adopt an
> overbearing approach. In this situation, superior power of
> whatever kind must be curbed. It appears variably in the rela-
> tionship of teacher to student, of jailer to prisoner, of physician
> to patient, and of scientist to subject. It can be "engineered" in a
> host of subtle ways. Whatever the mechanism, coercion nullifies
> consent.[4]

In the present study, subjects' ability to refuse was interfered with in
several ways. The most obvious but by no means the sole source of pressure
to participate came from subjects' reluctance to jeopardize their relationship with their physician. Perhaps because of their established relationship
with their physicians, *private* patients were particularly vulnerable to this
sort of pressure. The feared loss of the support of their physician was
highly threatening. Note that it was the established relationship, and not
the private physician per se, that was the operative factor here.

Clinic patients might seem to be potentially vulnerable to pressure because their ability to shop around for another source of health care is
limited. However, none of the clinic patients in the labor-induction study
indicated a belief that refusal to participate would have meant damage to
their relationships with the physicians or that they would have had to look
elsewhere for care if they refused. One subject did say, "I felt it might put
an edge between me and the doctors who suggested it in the first place [if I
had decided not to participate]." (#17, black, clinic) This statement,
however, was not given in response to a question about reasons for participation, and she gave other reasons for that; there was no indication that
this belief was an important reason for her participation. Of course, the
most obvious reason why fear of damage to their relationship with their
physicians was not a factor to clinic patients is that they did not have any
established relationship that could be threatened. As patients of the house
staff, they might never see the same doctor twice.

A second type of pressure to participate was lack of knowledge of options. This became a real source of pressure, in addition to being a matter
of ignorance, in situations where subjects believed that induction was
necessary and were told of no ways to have that induction other than
through the research.

In our discussion of subjects' decisions, it was pointed out that many subjects had no awareness of options. While the interview schedule did not
systematically cover the topic of options, subjects were asked what would
have been done if they had decided not to participate in the study. Almost
half (24 of 51) responded that they did not know what would have been
done, and the others responded with a variety of guesses. Five said they

would have been induced the regular way, 3 said they would have been induced at a later point, and 19 believed that they would have had to wait for natural labor. The latter group included a number of women who also believed that the health of their baby might be threatened by such a delay.

Looking at this from a slightly different perspective, data given to me by the research staff showed that labor-induction was medically indicated for 18 subjects. The remainder were elective inductions. Nevertheless, only five women believed that they could have been induced without delay if they had not wanted to participate. And in some of these cases, the belief was nothing more than a guess in response to a direct question from me. It is in this sense that women who believed they needed induction but did not know of any option other than the research were deprived of their freedom of choice.

The extent to which lack of options could prevent free choice in these cases is evident in the comments of several subjects:

R.   Wednesday I went in [to the clinic] and he talked to me about being 44 weeks pregnant and explained to me what could be happening inside—that fluids and the baby's afterbirth and everything could mingle, and that the baby could have a bowel movement inside and it could just go back into the baby's system—so they asked if they could take fluid from my stomach and see if it was clear or if it was cloudy. And they told me they would have to induce. So, then they took the fluid and everything and it was clear, and he talked to me about the study they are having on this. And he explained that there had only been 50 women or 51 that had used it in the last 4 or 5 years. And that Dr. P [the principal investigator] was the one who would give me the medication and everything. (#33, white, clinic)

I.   What did the doctor at the clinic say?

R.   He said I could be induced if I wanted. As a matter of fact, he said I didn't have too much choice because I was 2 weeks overdue. So he told me it would be best to go ahead and induce labor instead of just letting me sit around and try to get going on my own. (#25, black, clinic)

R.   When I went in he told me I was late and they don't like to have them go too long, you know. In case the baby has something wrong with it. He said I was small so they didn't want to let the baby grow too much. He put me on a diet. And he says that they have a new drug out and they wanted to try it if I was willing to go along with it. He said they can't make me take it, you know. So he set the date for me to come in . . . so that's how I'm in. (#11, white, clinic)

I. Why did you agree to participate?

R. I was under the impression that if I didn't there would be danger to the baby. Because of the weight gain, they said that you get complications and all the things that can happen. (#16, white, clinic)

These subjects, as well as some others, *believed that induction of labor was necessary* to the health of their baby; they had been told of the consequences of postdatism. However, *they were presented with only one way of being induced*—in research involving an experimental drug. They were not aware that nonexperimental inductions were routinely performed in cases in which there were medical indications.

Why did subjects not know that participation was optional? The obvious answer is that the topic was not covered in discussions or on the consent form. The comments of one subject who did know that her participation was optional are instructive:

I. If you had not agreed to be a subject, would you have come into the hospital anyway?

R. Yes.

I. You knew that?

R. Yes.

I. Did he tell you that explicitly or did you assume it?

R. No. I knew that I had a choice whether or not I wanted to be in it. I just thought "why not?"

I. Did he explicitly mention that you didn't have to? That you could come in for induction without being in the study? I'm curious.

R. Well, he didn't specifically mention it, but I knew from friends and relatives that have worked in the hospital section that research projects were a choice. You know, you had your choice as to whether or not you were going to participate.

I. Many people don't seem to be aware of that.

R. I think they neglect to mention it. They take if for granted that you know. I think that should be actually corrected. Because they take it for granted that people know they have a choice, and many people don't realize. (#30, white, clinic)

My findings clearly confirm her guess that many subjects did not realize that there was a choice when they were presented with a consent form. The most interesting thing about her comment was that she was able to deduce from the fact that research was involved that participation was voluntary and that there was a choice. Most subjects were not sophisticated enough about research and the investigator-subject relationship to make this deduction.

The idea that knowledge of options is necessary to informed consent is not a widely recognized one in the literature on human experimentation,[5] but the present study clearly indicates that it *should* be. Women who were convinced that induction was necessary and who knew of no way to be induced other than in the research were deprived of their freedom to refuse. That they may not have consciously felt that they had been constrained is beside the point. Although there was no medical reason for them to have been induced *in the study,* they had no real choice but to agree to participate.

A closely related problem was raised by the lack of knowledge of options among subjects who were committed, both mentally and through positive actions, to having labor induced *before* they learned of the research and its key elements. Many subjects made a decision to have their labor induced and acted on that decision (by making arrangements for the care of their other children and by being admitted to the hospital) before they learned that research was to be involved or what it required. In a very real sense these subjects were also deprived of the right to free choice of participation.

I. Why did you decide to participate?

R. Just because I am late. I should have had the baby the thirteenth [more than 2 weeks prior to the interview].

I. How were you told about the research? What did the doctor say?

R. Dr. V [clinic] told me . . . about being induced and everything. And at the time I went along with everything, because I figured I was late and I wanted to get it done and over with.

I. Did he mention that they were using a new drug?

R. Uh, I didn't know anything about the new drug or anything until I got to the hospital and then Dr. P [the principal investigator] explained the new drug and everything and what it would do.

I. Did Dr. V tell you there was research or did he just talk about being induced?

R. Just about being induced. Not particularly about it being a research project or anything . . . See, the reason I let them go ahead and induce labor and like I didn't know it was a research project really until I came to the hospital. It was explained a little bit but that's about it. Until I came here, and *then* I knew what was going on. So I didn't really have too much time to think about whether I should have or I shouldn't have it. (#14, white, clinic)

This subject went along with the situation as it unfolded, and was classified as a benefiting subject—even though her option of refusing to participate was limited—because she did not verbalize pressure as the main reason for her participation.

It may be remembered that three of the four unwilling subjects were among those who learned only in the labor room that an experimental drug was to be used. Two of them had been told before admission that they were to be "study" patients, but on learning in the labor room that an experimental drug was to be used they felt that it was too late for them to change their minds. At least two of them, however, became "difficult" subjects by raising a flood of questions after receiving the consent form. So the combination of circumstances whereby women learned of experimental drugs after they were heavily committed to having labor induced was definitely a factor that constrained them to participate, and, hence, represented an important failure in the consent process.

The fact that many subjects learned of the research (or at least about the key element—that an experimental drug was involved) for the first time in the labor room interfered with voluntary consent not only because these important revelations came after commitments to induction had been made. In addition, this factor was important because it prevented subjects from making a careful decision because of time constraints, and because it meant that subjects could not make their decision in a neutral setting.* Re-

* My findings show that the setting in which informed consent is to take place is of great importance in achieving valid consent. This obvious point has generally been overlooked in the literature on informed consent and in the regulation of human experimentation. Thus, for example, the need is not recognized for review committees to go beyond examining proposed consent forms to inquiring about the setting in which the form is to be given to subjects. However, even a clear consent form may be of little utility under unfavorable circumstances.

call the subject who described trying to discuss what she had learned from the consent form with her husband while one of the research nurses was present:

R.   If we were alone we maybe wouldn't have made such a rapid decision, you know. We could have been a little bit more open with each other. I just didn't feel quite comfortable discussing it with her. (#45, white, private)

In addition, this subject and others found that, because of the hospital's admission procedures, their husbands were filling out papers at the admitting office at the same time that the consent form (which was the first, and in some cases the sole information given to subjects) was presented in the labor room. In some cases, these circumstances effectively minimized or prevented, even if not by design of the researchers, husbands' participation in the decision, and deprived subjects of this source of advice.

The fact that the research often was presented for the first time to subjects after they had already been admitted was in and of itself an important factor limiting the freedom of women to refuse to participate. This aspect of the research, as will be discussed in the next section, had the additional consequence of contributing to the low level of understanding of the research that was common among subjects.

The final factor I wish to discuss is more diffuse. It appeared that many subjects may not have felt free to refuse because of the wide status gulf between them and physicians and because they felt they lacked the education to raise questions. I should hasten to point out that no subject said this. However, only high status patients raised the kind of sharp questions that might have been reasonable to raise. Furthermore, it was reflected in the fact that some low status patients seemed to agree to be subjects out of acquiescence rather than on this basis of any positive decision of their own.

This may have been partially because they were intimidated by being on the researchers' home ground where things that were strange and unfamiliar to subjects were routine to the research staff. Questions might have seemed likely only to further expose subjects' felt ignorance. Or they may have acquiesced because of the ubiquitous faith and trust in physicians we have already remarked on. Or it may be that some people did not know what was expected of them in this social situation. Most people ordinarily want to appear courteous and do not wish to offend, particularly when dealing with a respected figure. To some it may have seemed that raising questions would indicate mistrust, which might not be proper or which might bring sanctions.

Perhaps the acquiescence resulted partially from the sort of felt obligation described by the following committed subject:

R. Most people would probably have a tendency to feel that they were obligated since they were going through the clinic and receiving their medical treatment at very low costs anyway. They would have a tendency to feel that they were obligated to do this. It should be explained beforehand that there is no obligation as far as being a research experiment [sic]. (#30, white, clinic)

Although none of the clinic patients gave such reasons as the basis for their decision to volunteer, a mirror image of this view was given by a private patient who was not happy to learn, after her induction, that an experimental drug had been potentially involved. She was imagining the scenario if something were to go wrong with her baby as she said:

R. But it says nothing [on the consent form] about it being an experiment or research or anything.* But suppose we did have a problem. Just suppose. And they turn around and say, "You volunteered for this. This was experimental." I would get hysterical. I'd say, "I paid my doctor $500 to deliver a baby and I have to be subjected to an experiment?" But they have so many women. And I'm not downing them—don't misunderstand—but they have so many women that really wouldn't care and would volunteer, and they *prefer* going to the clinic, that could do this. (#29, white, private)

This subject is suggesting that it was somehow inappropriate to subject her to such risks because she had paid money for her care; such risks should be taken by those who "prefer" going to the clinic. I heard no comments from clinic patients that indicated that they shared this view. It may nevertheless be true that some clinic patients may have felt that it would not have been proper for them to raise objections because they were not going to pay for the careful attention they were receiving from very important, high status professionals.

I am suggesting that there is good reason, if not direct evidence, to believe that social distance between a highly educated professional and a poor patient with limited education is a significant barrier to a truly voluntary decision. This could perhaps be remedied by specific instruction to subjects that what is requested is voluntary, that they should express doubts and ask questions, and that they should not feel they have to take part if

* This, of course, was not entirely true since the words "experimental drugs" did appear on the form (see Appendix A).

they don't want to—for whatever reason—and that their relationship with those giving care to them will not be affected. Making all of these points explicit might or might not be sufficient. A further step would be the creation of a new ombudsmanlike role to be filled by a neutral person whose job it would be to help assure the voluntary and informed participation of subjects. Whether such a role is viable seems problematic. Not only would such a person be subject to pressures arising from his social status disadvantage vis-à-vis investigators; he would also presumably be an employee of the institution doing the research. How such a role could be located in career and authority structures is a further problem. Nevertheless, the concept of such a subject-assistant role might be worth investigating. An alternative would be to avoid using low status, poorly educated individuals as subjects except where direct therapeutic benefits are involved.

Deficiencies in Informing Subjects.   It has been pointed out that many labor-induction subjects (20 of 51) were not even aware of the research when their participation began, and that many more did not understand such key elements of the research as the possibility of unknown risks, the use of fetal monitoring equipment, the fact that additional blood samples were going to be taken, the double-blind aspect, and the fact that solicitation to study the newborn baby would result from participation. The presence of so many uninformed and partially informed subjects is a finding that must be examined.

A basic factor in accounting for the existence of uninformed and poorly informed subjects is the failure of the researchers to bridge educational and racial gaps. In the discussion of unaware subjects, we saw that the more dissimilar subjects were from the investigators, the less likely they were to be aware of the research before their participation began. In other words, the result of the procedures that were followed was that most highly educated subjects became at least aware of the research. However, the procedures followed did not communicate even at this rudimentary level with subjects with limited education. It must be stressed again that subjects cannot be blamed for this. The responsibility to inform subjects falls on investigators, and the existence of uninformed or poorly informed subjects means that that task was not adequately performed.

Interviews with subjects and familiarity with research procedures gained over several months of field work revealed several reasons why most labor-induction subjects had important gaps in their understanding of the research. There is no reason to think that these reasons are unique to that project, though how common the various factors might be in other projects is an open question.

First, no *one* person was assigned responsibility for seeing that the necessary information was conveyed to subjects. This is important because subjects came from several sources and had seen different physicians prior to coming into contact with the researchers for the first time in the labor room.

I. What doctors did you see prior to coming into the hospital?

R. Oh God, I can't think of their names.

I. A lot of them?

R. Yes. (#21, black, clinic)

R. He told me yesterday that he would induce my labor but he didn't say nothing, you know, about the study or . . .

I. What doctor was that?

R. Dr. V [clinic].

I. Then he called you Monday?

R. The nurse called me Monday morning . . . And when I came in they just started getting me ready to induce labor. They didn't, you know, say anything about being a study.

I. Then what? Did they give you a form to sign or did they explain first or what?

R. No. She gave me a form and told me to read it and sign it. So I read it and said, "Well, might as well go ahead with it." So I signed it.

I. Did they explain more than what was on the form, or was that all?

R. No. They didn't explain.

I. Have you seen any doctors yet this morning?

R. Yes, Dr. P [principal investigator].

I. Is he the one that hooked you up and everything?

R. Yes.

I. Did he tell you anything about what he was doing and why and things like that?

R. No. He just said that he was ready to get started. I guess he figured they had already told me. (#10, black, clinic)

These comments, particularly the last one by an unaware subject with less than a high school education, graphically illustrate how responsibility for informing subjects can be neglected when several people are involved with subjects at different points. It is easy to imagine everyone assuming that somebody else had informed (or would inform) subjects about the research.

Since physicians other than the researchers had the initial role in involving subjects in the research, the instructions under which they performed this role are of interest. The principal investigator told me that he had held a meeting with the residents on the house staff at the beginning of the research and had asked them to inform prospective subjects about the research before sending them in to be induced. Nevertheless, about two-thirds of the subjects coming from the clinics indicated that they knew nothing about the research qua research until they were handed the consent form in the labor room (if they even realized then). One reason for this was probably the residents' use of euphemisms such as "new drug" and "study patient," a factor to be discussed below.

With regard to private physicians, the principal investigator said that he felt it was not his place to suggest how they should inform their patients. Not all of these physicians even chose to inform them, although some private patients received detailed explanations. Both private physicians and clinic physicians may have assumed that a complete explanation would be given after women had reached the labor room. Almost half of the private patients (8 of 17) did not know before admission that research was to be involved in their induction.

Likewise, the two investigators themselves could have easily assumed that patients were being informed. The principal investigator had given instructions to the house staff, and at the time of the investigators' usual first contact with subjects, the subjects were already in the labor room. Preliminary preparations had been completed, a signed consent form was nearby, and subjects were awaiting the start of the drug infusion. An investigator entering the room might well conclude that the subject had already been informed. Even without reaching this conclusion, it would hardly have seemed appropriate to begin an explanation of the research at that point.

All of this suggests that often subjects could participate without having received any information about the research from a physician. This was in fact indicated by subjects' responses to several questions. Although all patients saw a physician prior to admission, 31 (of 50 reporting) did not know research was to be involved before they were admitted. When asked, "Who did you talk to connected with the study?" only 18 of 46 reporting said that they talked to the principal investigator, and 8 said that they talked to his co-investigator. A few of the higher status patients reported having demanded to talk to a doctor after they were given the consent form, but many subjects perhaps did not feel secure enough to make this kind of demand. So physicians had a very uneven role in giving information to subjects; many different doctors were involved before admission, and after admission the investigators often did not take an active informational role.

The only constants in the process of giving subjects information about the research were the research nurses (all but one subject reported talking to the research nurses before the drug infusion began) and the consent form. The importance of the nurses in this regard is reflected in the subjects' responses to a question concerning who had told them most about the study before their participation had begun. Eleven subjects said that the nurses told them most; 5 said they learned most from the principal investigator, two from the co-investigator, 7 from physicians on the house staff, and 5 from private physicians.

The two research nurses seemed to have taken the responsibility for getting consent forms signed almost by default, partially because they had the first actual contact with subjects after their admission. The principal investigator gave convenience as the main reason why the nurses performed this task, and said that he had not given them any special instructions because they had long experience as research nurses. Although they took responsibility for getting a signature on the consent form, it was not clear how much responsibility they felt for *informing* subjects. (Given the fact that all subjects signed the form but many were not informed, the distinction between getting a signature on the form and informing subjects is an important one.) It is also not clear whether the nurses were really aware that most subjects knew little or nothing about the project prior to their admission.

For whatever reason, an explanation did not necessarily accompany the consent form in the labor room. This was indicated by the subjects who reported being given the form with the instructions to "read this and sign it," and it resulted in the large number of subjects who were not aware of what they had signed. Fourteen of 47 responding subjects said that less than 5 minutes had been spent in explaining the study to them, and another 9 said that the explanation had consumed less than 15 minutes.

The nurses' failure to inform subjects was not due to their reluctance to talk about the research with subjects. *After* the drug infusion had begun, the nurses talked with subjects about the research during the long day that they would spend together. Many subjects commented enthusiastically about how much they had learned from the nurses during the day and how much they had felt a part of the whole procedure. The importance of the nurses in this regard was reflected in subjects' responses to the question: "Overall—both before and during the study—who explained or told you the most about the study?" Subjects' answers were distributed as follows:

Research nurses   19
Principal investigator   4
Co-investigator   3
House staff   2
Private physician   2
Consent form   2
Interviewer (author)   8

From these responses and from additional comments from the subjects, it is apparent that nurses imparted much information throughout the day while subjects were in labor. However, several factors worked against detailed, unsolicited explanations by the nurses at the time the consent form was presented to subjects. This goes right to the heart of the problem caused by the delegation of the consent-seeking task.

First, these nurses were supposed to get the consent form signed, but they had no clear responsibility for seeing that subjects received a full explanation. Second, getting subjects' signatures on consent forms was only one of many tasks and procedures that had to be carried out by the nurses prior to the starting of the drug infusion by one of the investigators. The longer it took to perform these tasks the longer would be their day, since the nurses stayed until after delivery (up to 14 hours among the subjects interviewed) or until the end of labor (the drug infusion was stopped after 10 hours, but labor could continue for some time, even for those who failed to deliver). Of course, some labors were quite short. Nevertheless there were strong incentives for the research nurses to be as brisk as possible with the pre–infusion tasks, of which the consent form was one.

Third, and most importantly, it was the nurses' job to *assist the investigator.* This was done in innumerable ways. Causing difficulty with research subjects would have been inconsistent with such a role. Certainly the nurses would not wish to be responsible for causing a subject to refuse to participate after being admitted to the hospital. An occasional subject became upset in the labor room upon learning of the study or of the fact that experimental drugs were involved. These situations could be awkward and difficult to handle, so there was ample incentive to keep everything under control.

The ways that matters were kept under control, however, mitigated against subjects' being informed adequately. Perhaps the primary method of maintaining this control was to treat things connected with the research as being routine in nature. For example, certain words were avoided. As already noted, one of the research nurses warned me against using the word "experiment." I was also told by one of the research nurses that "the word 'research' is never used" around the subjects. Furthermore, as previously mentioned, the experimental drugs were always called "new drugs" by the professionals, by subjects, and by me. One had the feeling that the situation vis-à-vis subjects was delicate and that one had to be very circumspect in making references to the research. Words that were possibly emotionally charged were thus avoided in favor of terms that neither aroused subjects nor, in many cases, conveyed the essential nature of the matter to them.

Several unaware subjects commented on their misunderstanding of the various euphemisms that were used:

R. When he said a "study patient," I assumed that he was talking about inducement and this was how he referred to it. I didn't realize that it was anything more than that . . . Actually my sister's husband said that a study case would be like research. So *he* was fully aware of what was involved. I said, "Oh, no. I have my *own* doctor, and why would *that* be?" Usually a clinic case would volunteer to be a study case, you know. Right? (#29, white, private)

I. Did they tell you anything about using a new drug to induce labor? Did you know anything about that?

R. They was telling me about that they had a new drug they were using.

I. Did you know it was a research drug, or . . .

R. No. (#42, black, clinic)

I. Is it correct that you really weren't aware about the research until I started talking about it?

R. No, she didn't mention anything about research, but I'm sure she mentioned that it's a new drug. I'm sure. (#44, black, clinic)

R. They didn't tell me no more than they explained to me when I made the appointment. That it was . . . uh . . . well, it was said that it was a new medicine, a new drug.

I. Did you realize that meant research?

R. No. (#50, black, clinic)

Consistent with the pervasive use of euphemisms was the apparently offhand manner in which the consent form was presented to subjects, the unspoken suggestion being that it was merely routine. "Sign this and we can get started," one subject reported being told. The impact of the routinization of the consent form presentation can be seen in the following comments, all from unaware subjects:

R. And when I came in they just started getting me ready to induce labor. They didn't, you know, say anything about being a study.

I. Then what? Did they give you a form to sign or did they explain first, or what?

R. No. She gave me a form and told me to read it and sign it. So I read it and said, "Well, might as well go ahead with it." So I signed it.

I. Did they explain more than what was on the form, or was that all?

R. No. They didn't explain.

I. Why did you agree after you read the paper? Any particular reason?

R. Why did I sign the paper for the drugs?

I. Yes?

R. Well, I figured to get me started they would have to give me a drug to induce it. You have to sign a paper for it. Usually you have to sign for medications and stuff they give you. (#10, black, clinic)

I. How much time did they spend explaining the study and discussing it with you?

R. They didn't explain.

I. They just gave you the paper to read and sign?

R. The nurse brought the paper. The nurse did.

I. Did you ask questions about it?

R. No. She told me to read it and I read it.

I. Then you signed it?

R. Uh-hum. (#18, black, clinic)

I. You say that you did not know they were using a new drug to induce labor?

R. No, I had no idea that that was what they were using.

I. Did they have you sign something when you came in?

R. Yeah, they had me sign the paper like they always do stating that, you know, if I need any medication or something like this here it's all right for them to give it to me. And stuff like that.

I. And you didn't sign a paper that said . . .

R. None that said anything about a drug that's supposed to induce labor. I didn't even know that that's what that was. They just had the tube sitting on the machine and said, "Now that's your medicine." That's all. (#06, black, clinic)

The appearance that everything was routine was helped by the fact that the research consent form was the second of two consent forms signed by subjects (the first one was truly routine). In addition, the research was outwardly similar to a normal labor induction, particularly at the beginning. At the beginning of induction the only difference from a nonresearch induction—the drug being infused—was not visible. (By contrast, the requirements of the starvation-abortion study were of a more obviously nonroutine nature. It would have been far more difficult—though not impossible if one recalls the earlier described case of the woman who seemed to want to believe the starvation would result in a greater chance of a successful abortion—to have involved subjects in a project requiring 3 days of starvation without their knowing that something not dictated solely by therapeutic considerations was involved.)

All of this suggests that the danger of leaving subjects relatively or completely uninformed is heightened when an investigator gives the consent responsibility to a subordinate. Because of the nature of superordinate-subordinate relationships, the tendency is for the subordinate to perform the visible aspects of the task (getting a signed form) at the expense of the less tangible task of seeing that the subjects have the necessary understanding. This is particularly true in situations in which the subordinate might fear that full disclosure might alarm the subject and jeopardize the chances of "getting the consent."

Also undoubtedly responsible for so many subjects signing the form without knowing that research was involved was the fact that subjects with no prior knowledge of the research were given the form in the labor room. As previously noted, this interfered with their ability freely to deliberate about whether to participate. The labor room was not only a poor place for newly informed subjects to deliberate about participating; it was also obviously a poor place to *inform* subjects. Thirty-one subjects did not know they were to be in a research study when they were admitted and reached the labor room; of these, 20 never did find out until their participation was underway or was complete, although they all signed the consent form.

This becomes more understandable when one remembers that patients were entering the hospital at 7:00 A.M. prepared to be induced and prepared to sign the necessary forms. Their attention was focused on the task at hand, which was the culmination of months of waiting and planning. Hence, they were not in a good position to give careful attention to anything other than the job ahead of them. As one unaware subject remarked:

R. I talked to the doctor who put this stuff in [indicated the IV equipment], and he explained to me about what they are trying to do.

I. Do you remember what he told you?

R. No, I was just concentrating on having the baby, and getting it over with. (#06, black, clinic)

The comments of the following subject illustrate both the problem of presenting the consent form as routine and the disinterest of subjects in such matters at that particular time:

I. I understand that they might be using a new drug in your induction. Did they say anything about that?

R. No, they didn't say anything.

I. Did they give you a piece of paper that explained anything about being induced?

R. No.

I. I just want to be sure about this because on some of the people having labor induced that I have talked to they are using a new drug. But they didn't say anything about that or give you a form to sign or anything?

R. No. [pause] I had to sign a form though, but I didn't feel like reading it right then. She told me it was just so that they had my agreement to go through with it. (#21, black, clinic)

Because only cursory, euphemistic verbal explanations were given to labor-induction subjects, the consent form assumed major importance in informing them. By contrast, in the starvation-abortion study relatively complete oral explanations were necessary in order to successfully gain women's agreement to undergo a 3-day fast, and the consent form itself was of much less importance. The researchers in the starvation-abortion study were very casual about when the form was signed; it was usually *not* signed before a woman began her fast, but was always signed before discharge. However, in that study the consent form was truly a formality. It did not play an important role in *informing* subjects. In the labor-induction study, however, giving subjects information about the research did not play the same role of enhancing the probability of subjects' agreement to participate. In fact, since the most hesitant women were among the best informed subjects, giving information might have had just the opposite effect. Thus, many subjects reported getting little information other than that on the consent form. The consent form provided the only information that was systematically given to all subjects, and thus was obviously an important document in the consent process in the labor-induction study.

However, the usefulness of the consent form in informing labor-induction subjects was somewhat limited by three factors. First and most important, it was not necessarily supplemented with verbal explanations. Second, its nature and purpose were misunderstood by many subjects. Many thought it was just one of the hospital's routine forms that had to be signed in order for a woman to have her baby there. At the other extreme were two highly educated subjects who interpreted the form as a "release" that would absolve the hospital and the researchers of any responsibility for untoward effects of the experimental drugs. Even though they were assured that this was not the form's purpose, they both ended up as unwilling subjects.

Part of the reason for misinterpretation of the consent form, particularly by those who thought it was routine, was its somewhat euphemistic heading (standard at the institution): "Patient Consent Form for Participation in a Clinical Investigation." While the term "clinical investigation" might not carry the negative connotations that are perhaps associated with the terms "experiment" or "research," it did not convey very much to many patients, particularly to those of low educational levels. (The consent form is reprinted in Appendix A.)

The third limitation of the consent form was that it was not complete. The fact that several blood samples were to be taken was not mentioned. It also failed to mention the planned 6-hour observation (with blood samples and X rays) of the baby, which was usually presented to the subject for her consent during labor or shortly after delivery. Although a separate investigator was conducting that study, it was being done because an experimental drug was being used to induce labor. This was a serious shortcoming of the form, since many of the women going into labor expressed more concern about the health of their baby than about anything else.

Perhaps the most important omission on the consent form (and the whole consent procedure itself) was that no reference was made to alternatives to participation. As was mentioned earlier, even most of the aware subjects were unclear as to what were their alternatives to participation.

The complexity of the informed consent issue is reflected in the many factors that were related to the existence of many completely uninformed and only partially informed labor-induction subjects. The consent problems discussed thus far resulted from the procedures that were followed in acquiring subjects and in "getting their consent." In the final section of this chapter, we discuss a different type of factor, one that involved the role expectations that were brought by many subjects to the research situation.

Lack of Understanding of the Research Subject Role. The final main factor interfering with informed consent is perhaps the least specific to the particular research projects described in this book. It flows from the lack of sophistication many people have about basic differences between the doctor-patient relationship and the researcher-subject relationship. In particular, subjects' lack of awareness of the special requirements of the subject role is an important barrier to informed consent. Before looking at evidence from my study, let us briefly consider some aspects of these two role relationships.

The doctor-patient relationship is, of course, quite familiar, and the patient role is deeply institutionalized. In his classic formulation, Parsons outlined four aspects of the institutionalized expectations system relative to the sick role.[6] Crucial here is the fourth element, the patient's "obligation to seek technically competent help, namely, in the most usual case, that of a physician and to cooperate with him in the process of trying to get well."[7] And in discussing the collectively-oriented nature of the patient-physician relationship, Parsons says:

> It is true that the patient has a very obvious self-interest in get-
> ting well . . . But once he has called in a physician the attitude is
> clearly marked, that he has assumed the obligation to cooperate
> with that physician in what is regarded as a common task. The
> obverse of the physicians' obligation to be guided by the welfare
> of the patient is the latter's obligation to "do his part" to the
> best of his ability.[8]

But what of the situation where the physician has another interest, namely research, instead of or in addition to his interest in the patient's welfare? One would hope that this would never preclude an interest in the patient's welfare. But, warns Louis Jaffe,

> even where the experiment may benefit the patient, the phy-
> sician-investigator may develop an interest in the experiment
> which qualifies his devotion to his patient. This situation may be
> more likely if the patient is a charity or semi-charity patient, and
> there has been no pre-existing personal relationship between phy-
> sician and patient.[9]

Accordingly, where research interests are present, current ethical standards dictate that a subject's participation must be based on informed consent.

Distinctions between the doctor-patient relationship and the researcher-subject relationship are frequently offered in the literature on human experimentation. It has been pointed out, for example, that the "physician *accepts* patients and is concerned with their welfare; the investigator *selects* subjects—problems as well as individuals—and, while responsive to the patient's interest, is more concerned with solving the scientific problem."[10] This matter of intended benefit is mentioned by other writers as well. Blumgart, for example, says:

> The doctor-patient relationship has the welfare of the patient as
> its primary objective and may be characterized as a therapeutic
> alliance. The experimenter-subject relationship, on the other

hand, has the discovery of new knowledge as its primary objective and may be termed a scientific alliance.[11]

The differences between the doctor-patient relationship and the researcher-
subject relationship were given at least quasi-legal status by the New York
Board of Regents in the Brooklyn Jewish Chronic Disease Hospital case of
the early 1960s. Live cancer cells were injected into 22 elderly patients
without their knowledge.[12] A basic principle advanced by the Board in its
hearings was that "the physician, when he is acting as experimenter, cannot
claim those rights of doctor-patient relationships that do permit him, in a
therapeutic situation, to withhold information when he judges it to be in the
best interests of his patient."[13]

All of this suggests that the relationship between subject and researcher,
and the normative expectations attached to that relationship, differ from
the physician-patient relationship, because whereas Parsons talked of the
patient's "obligation to do his part," the research subject is not considered
to have such an obligation. Interestingly, in the present study almost all
subjects (more than 80 percent) responded to a direct question by saying
that one does *not* have an "obligation to cooperate" where research is involved, but that such participation is a purely voluntary matter. Many of
these subjects were not aware that their permission *had* been requested, and
that they had reacted to this request in a manner more appropriate to the
physician-patient relationship by cooperating as they would if treatment
were being suggested by a therapist. That, of course, is the point that
concerns us in this discussion.

As an aside, Beecher has argued that it is dangerous for the physician to
adopt a different role vis-à-vis research subjects, because researchers might
come to feel that the ethical obligations that are held to be valid for the
doctor-patient relationship do not apply if the person has given his consent
to participate in research. He argues that "the doctor-investigator cannot
be any more neglectful of the interest of a group of individuals under his
responsibility in the laboratory, for the sake of science, than he is of one
patient in his consulting room who comes for therapy."[14] One does not
have to take issue with that principle to argue that it is necessary to the
success of informed consent for the *subject* to realize that there is something about the research situation that differs from the usual encounters
between patient and physician, encounters in which many people place
themselves in the physician's hands and follow whatever he might recommend. What differs in the research situation is that the researcher's
interests go beyond the individual subject; the subject thus has additional
responsibilities involving a decision about whether or not to allow something involving his body or mind to be done. If the subject does not accept

his responsibility to make such a decision (and to raise whatever questions may be necessary), then our current methods of protecting subjects in part by giving them to the opportunity to refuse to participate in research fail to operate properly. This happened in the present study.

Informed consent is obviously not adequate, in and of itself, to protect subjects' interests. Review committees that make judgments about whether the risks of a proposed project are justified by the potential benefits, and that have the technical expertise to make sure that all prudent safety procedures are followed have an important role. But as things stand, these committees also assume that prospective subjects, by raising questions and by making independent judgments, will take a role in protecting themselves.

As we have seen, however, many people who enter the hospital as patients do not recognize the basic differences between therapy and research. Specifically, many potential subjects do not understand the expectation that they will look out for their own interests when presented with the decision to take part in research, nor the fact that researchers have interests that transcend the health or illness of any particular subject. In reality, both scientific interests and career interests are involved. With regard to the former, the eminent biomedical scientist Dr. Szent-Gyorgyi has stated:

> Desire to alleviate suffering [is] of small value in research—such a person should be advised to work for a charity. Research wants egotists, damn egotists, who seek their own pleasure and satisfaction, but find it in solving the puzzles of nature.[15]

The career interests of investigators* have been well described by Henry Beecher:

> Every young physician knows that he will never be promoted to a tenure post, to a professorship in a major medical school, unless he has proved himself as an investigator. If the ready availability of money for conducting research is added to this fact, one can see how great are the pressures on ambitious young physicians.[16]

None of the subjects I interviewed recognized these career interests of researchers.

* The impact of career contingencies on investigators' ethics and behavior is a central focus of the analysis presented by Bernard Barber, John J. Lally, Julia Loughlin Makarushka, and Daniel Sullivan in *Research on Human Subjects: Problems of Social Control in Medical Experimentation,* (New York: Russell Sage, 1973.) See particularly Chs. 4 and 5.

In the ideal typical situation, the physician as therapist has a long-term interest in the patient and only a transitory interest in any particular episode or treatment that might be used. The researcher's interest in the subject lasts only for the duration of a particular experiment episode. However, his interest in the treatment both precedes his contact with the subject and remains after that contact has ended. The practicing physician fulfills and attains professional stature by his success in dealing with patients' problems; thus an unsuccessful attempt at inducing labor would, for example, be detrimental to the private physician as well as to his patient, because that physician depends on his reputation among patients for continued professional success. But an unsuccessful attempt at inducing labor may be of benefit to the researcher in that it may teach him a great deal. In fact, to the extent that his professional reputation may be influenced by his demonstration that one drug fails less often than another drug, failure among a certain proportion of his subjects might be seen as consistent with his career interests which depend on the success or failure of his research rather than on his ability to satisfy patients.

Two questions might be asked to determine whether a subject recognizes the special aspects of the researcher-subject relationship. Is the subject aware that a researcher has personal and career interests that go beyond immediate patient care? And does he abdicate his right of consent by leaving the decision in the hands of the researcher? By both measures the subjects in the present study proved unsophisticated about research and the role of the research subject, and this seriously undermined the consent process. Let us examine each question.

To determine subjects' consciousness of researchers' career interests, subjects were asked two questions. Among the fixed-response questions concerning subject reasons for participating in the labor-induction study was the question, "Did you believe that it would help the researchers if you participated? If so, in what way?" Of the 26 subjects who indicated their belief that their participation would help the researchers, not one showed awareness that the help would be in terms of his *career*. Instead, most subjects talked of helping the researchers advance science or gain knowledge, as in these comments:

R.   What way would it help the researchers? Well, it might give them more clues as to how it reacts. You know, anything that they are using. I think it helps. (#12, white, private)

R.   I would think they could find out a lot more of what goes on in labor with the baby. (#40, white, private)

R. [It would help the researchers] just by furthering their knowledge of the labor mechanism. (#46, white, private)

R. The more research done on an object, the more you can accomplish. (#30, white, clinic)

R. I believe everybody who participates helps some because then they can get whatever their scale would be . . . the more they get the better it would be for everybody concerned. (#07, white, clinic)

R. [It would help the researchers] to learn more about what's happening, about what's going on. (#14, white, clinic)

R. It just gave them another day, another person to compare. (#22, white, private)

R. I would be one more guinea pig that they wouldn't have to get. (#16, white, clinic)

R. I knew that if they were trying a new drug they would like to find as many subjects as they could. (#17, black, clinic)

Twenty-four subjects gave similar responses. The other two responded in terms of helping the researchers learn how to better treat other patients.

I. In what way would it help the researchers?

R. Help them to help other people. Other women, I should say. (#41, white, clinic)

R. They might find out something different or something new that might help out in some other case or something. (#28, black, clinic)

On this first item, asked only of aware subjects because it concerned reasons for participation in research, subjects showed no recognition of the fact that researchers have career interests that differ from the usual practicing physician.

The second item was asked of all subjects. After being asked whether subjects or future patients generally benefit the most from medical research, subjects were asked, "How about researchers—do they benefit?" Of the 46 subjects responding, only 2 mentioned that the researchers would benefit from research in terms of their professional careers. Most responses were similar to those just quoted. More than half of those responding answered in terms such as "it will help them learn more," "Well, they gain the experience and the knowledge," "They get their information and therefore they can make their evaluations." About one-sixth of those responding mentioned that the researchers would benefit by being better able to help their patients.

R.   Probably they will learn a little more that will help them in the long run with future patients. (#28, black, clinic)

R.   Maybe they'll know more for the next patient. (#16, white, clinic)

R.   Well, if anyone were coming in under the same circumstances they would know what to do. (#47, black, clinic)

Four subjects saw the researcher as benefiting because of the satisfaction of inner needs:

R.   Well, in the first place they would feel that they have achieved something by inventing the thing in the first place. And I'm sure that they feel just as proud as the person they used it on in the first place. (#17, black, clinic)

R.   Gratification of their humanitarian impulses. (#13, white, private)

R.   This is their particular field and if you engage in research you have your own reasons for your interests. It could be spiritual. (#19, white, private)

R.   Well, through their patients I guess they get satisfaction, but I don't see where they get much other benefit. (#33, white, clinic)

The two labor-induction subjects who showed an awareness of the researcher's career interests said:

R. Well, I'm sure that drug is never going to help Dr. P [principal investigator], but it would benefit him, I suppose, if he were to make some great discovery. Financially benefit him. (#04, white, private)

R. Only if they can make a discovery or make a great contribution so they become famous. (#46, white, private)

Even here, though, subjects were thinking in the glamorous terms of a great discovery rather than in the more realistic terms of whether the investigator's promotion to the next academic rank depends on his having a certain number of research papers published in certain journals. Considering researchers' need for subjects in those terms would perhaps increase the likelihood that one would be very careful about agreeing to be a subject.

This lack of awareness of researchers' interests was, I believe, partially responsible for the faulty consent process in the labor-induction study. Patients reacted to the researchers as they would to any other physician, that is, they followed a physician's wishes without question. This is hardly an adequate basis for informed consent in research.

The second indicator of subjects' lack of awareness of requirements of the subject's role is whether they wanted to take part in the decision that involved them in research. Apparently many people are accustomed to giving their physician total freedom to treat them as he sees fit. This type of physician-patient relationship was described well by the subject who said:

R. . . . if my doctor says, "Well, I feel this is what you should do," I would have done it. You know, without doubt if that's what he told me to do. I mean, any person not being a doctor would feel the same way. If they are going to a specialist and he says, "Well, take this vitamin," you take it. (#29, white, private)

This type of response to a physician's wishes may be appropriate (whether or not it is desirable) to the patient role as Parsons described it. It is not appropriate to the research situation in which the subject supposedly makes his own decision, however. That the researcher often is the sole source of information on which this decision is based may also interfere with a subject's ability to make a free decision.

Responses from subject after subject in the labor-induction study indicate that they participated because that was how the physician (researcher) wanted it done. In medical matters, the physician had the answers.

I. When you were asked to participate—did it occur to you to say no?

R. No, because I figured the doctor knows best. (#20, black, clinic)

I. Why did you decide to participate?

R. That was the way they wanted to do it. I wasn't going to argue with them. They know what they are doing, I guess. (#31, white, private)

R. The doctors felt that was what I should do, so I went. (#42, black, clinic)

R. I think a doctor always gives you his way of thinking—what's best for you. And if that's part of a study, then that's the way for you. (#33, white, clinic)

A closely related response, which clearly shows a fundamental lack of understanding of researchers' needs for volunteers, was given by subjects who indicated that they agreed because they assumed they would not have been asked if they did not need the particular method involved.

I. Why did you agree to participate?

R. I figured they knew what they were doing. There had to be a reason to ask me. (#05, white, clinic)

R. I knew they thought I should [participate]. Otherwise they would never have taken me down there [to the labor room] in the first place. (#17, black, clinic)

R. Last time, three and a half years ago, I was worried about that peridural they gave me and wouldn't go through with it. Then the doctor finally talked me into it, and I took it. And I'm glad I took it. So this time when he went and asked me about this I figured it was the same as last time, and they were going to help me out, so "good, go right ahead." (#11, white, clinic)

These subjects apparently could not conceive of research in which there was no benefit to the subject, or of a researcher asking a subject to participate because he needed a subject.

All of these responses show a lack of a fundamental understanding of the nature of research, the nature of the researcher-subject relationship, and the expectation that the subject will provide a measure of self-protection by exercising some degree of judgment regarding his own participation. Data from the present study offer some clues as to the reasons for this lack of understanding.

First, there was a lack of previous experience with research. Only the one faculty patient had previous experience in biomedical research. This had been during the present pregnancy and had been highly therapeutic in nature, dealing with the Rh difficulties in her pregnancy. (She did not define this as research and, in fact, responded negatively to my question concerning previous research experience.) Eight other subjects had taken part in social or psychological research while college students. Although most subjects lacked any previous research experience, nothing was done in the present situation to educate them to their responsibility in the decision process.

Second, many subjects were not informed that the physicians who were going to induce their labor were researchers, and there was nothing to distinguish the researchers from other physicians except the additional consent form. A college educated private patient told of her difficulty in figuring out who the researchers were and what was their role:

R. I didn't really talk to [the researchers] before the induction was started. They just kind of came in and got things going. And that was . . . I was trying to figure out how they really fit into the picture, you know, at that point. And I thought maybe there were certain doctors that did the induction, you know, that Dr. D [her private physician] didn't do it, but other doctors did. (#36, white, private)

As we have noted, the procedure itself appeared normal, unlike the quite apparent research aspect in the starvation-abortion study. Since the procedure itself offered subjects few clues that research was being done, they related to the researchers as they would have to any physician giving them treatment.

Finally, due to the previously described high level of faith in medicine verbalized by several subjects, the degree of independence implied by the concept of making one's own decision may have been unthinkable:

R. I figured that if the doctor's didn't know what they were doing they wouldn't ask me to come in. (#21, black, clinic)

Another potential factor is the possible role confusion that may be created when a physician who has established a therapist-patient relationship asks his patient to take part in research. This factor was not important in my study because the researchers did not have a previously established therapeutic relationship with the subjects.

Having a private physician can either enhance or diminish the chances of free consent taking place. If it is clear to a subject that his cooperation is desired by researchers (other than his own physician) who are in need of volunteers, then the subject has in his own physician a trusted source of medical advice. A number of private patients reported that their private physician played this kind of a role in the present study:

R. ... he really believed in it—my doctor did—and I figured as long as he felt it was safe I was willing to go along with it. (#12, white, private)

R. I'm sure Dr. M wouldn't subject us to something like this unless it was completely safe. We have a lot of confidence in him. (Husband of #45, white, private)

R. I really based my decision on the fact that he recommended it—Dr. D. I have absolute faith in his judgment, and I figure that he wouldn't recommend something that he felt would be harmful. (#32, white, private)

While this kind of faith in one's physician can be supportive in a situation requiring an important decision, a patient's critical ability might be impaired by his perception of his physician's desires, particularly if the patient does not understand that an option is involved. The comments of these and other private patients (and of some clinic patients as well) indicate that many people hold a somewhat inflexible view of what a physician might ask a patient to do. The possibility that the physician might ask a patient to do something that is not for the patient's benefit does not arise.

R. I don't think a doctor is going to ask a person unless he feels that they themselves [the subjects] are going to benefit. Why would my family physician call me or tell me in a visit, "I'd like you to participate," unless he felt that this would benefit me? (#24, white, private)

It is of great importance, therefore, for a physician to make sure the patient clearly understands the nature of the situation when he is asking the patient to do something for extratherapeutic reasons. The concept of physician is strongly linked in people's minds with the concept of therapist, who has only the patient's interests in mind. It may be difficult for the patient to shift gears into the subject role with a physician with whom he has established the therapist-patient relationship.

A final, telling indicator of subjects' lack of preparedness for assuming the responsibilities of the subject role came in their responses to the question, "On the basis of your experience, what factors would you say one should consider before deciding to be a research subject? What would you advise a friend to find out about if she was asked to take part in some medical research?" Most subjects who could respond gave only general, vague answers such as, "I would advise them to find out everything they could about it." Twenty-seven subjects gave such answers. But, perhaps surprisingly, even with probing, most subjects did not mention any of the types of factors that might seem obvious. Twenty-three said they should find out about risks, 13 said they should find out how the research might be of benefit to them, 8 mentioned learning about the scientific importance of the research, 2 said potential subjects should learn whether pain and discomfort were going to be involved, and 1 mentioned that they should learn whether the research would involve any inconvenience.

All of this suggests that researchers must take the active role in making the relevant information available to subjects. It cannot be left to the subject to raise the proper questions. People who basically trust physicians and only conceive of them in the therapist role may be unprepared to assume an important self-protection role in the research situation.

NOTES

1. Henry K. Beecher, *Research and the Individual* (Boston: Little, Brown, 1970), p. 18.
2. Jay Katz, *Experimentation with Human Beings* (New York: Russell Sage, 1973), pp. 523–524.
3. Ibid., pp. 523–608.
4. Beecher, op. cit., p. 30.
5. The need to specify alternatives is, however, explicitly mentioned in the definition of the elements of informed consent in the *Institutional Guide to DHEW Policy on Protection of Human Subjects* (1971), p. 7.
6. Talcott Parsons, *The Social System* (New York: Free Press, 1964 [1951]), pp. 433–465.
7. Ibid., p. 437.

8. Ibid., p. 438.

9. Louis L. Jaffe, "Law as a System of Social Control," *Daedalus,* 98 (Spring 1969), 417.

10. Beecher, op. cit., p. 79. Beecher is paraphrasing an earlier statement by Irving Ladimer.

11. Herrman L. Blumgart, "The Medical Framework for Viewing the Problem of Human Experimentation," *Daedalus,* 98 (Spring 1969), 248.

12. See Chapter One, p. 00.

13. Bernard Barber, "Experimenting with Humans," *The Public Interest* (Winter 1967), 93.

14. Beecher, op. cit., p. 90.

15. Katz, *Experimentation with Human Beings,* p. 648.

16. Beecher, op. cit., p. 16.

CHAPTER NINE

SUMMARY AND IMPLICATIONS

In this final chapter I want to examine some of the implications of my findings. The discussion, which is partly based on subjects' own reflections about their experiences in research, is preceded by a summary of some of the major findings of this study.

1. While the use of human subjects is necessary to much medical research, subjects are sometimes able to use research to meet their own needs while they are being used by the researchers. An interesting aspect of the labor-induction study was that some subjects *used the research,* while other subjects were only *used by the research.* This was largely a function of whether the physician who recruited them for the study was a private physician or a member of the house staff.

There were several indications that private physicians used the research for their patients' medical benefit or to meet patients' stated desires of having their babies at the earliest possible time. Many private patients knew why they had been asked to participate and indicated that they had expressed a desire for the earliest possible delivery. They were grateful for the chance to participate because it met their own felt needs. In this sense, their physician was acting as their agent in involving them in the research. This was also reflected by the extent to which private patients reported turning to their physicians for advice and assurance in their participation decisions.

The relationship between the private physician and his patient was not without its dangers, however. Some private patients were unwilling subjects; they feared that their established relationship with their physician might be threatened by their refusal to do what they felt their physician wanted them to do—that is, participate in the labor-induction study. An established doctor-patient relationship can clearly interfere with a genuine consent process. Thus, the doctor-patient relationship is not always a mighty protector of the patient as research subject.

While private physicians acted largely as their patients' agents (a characterization contaminated by the unknown role played by the friendship and professional interlocks between these physicians and the investigators), the house staff was apparently acting as the researchers' agents. Thus, clinic patients, who were overrepresented among the subject population, were more likely to be "used" by the research than to use the research. For example, it was to the house staff that calls for subjects went on mornings when clinics were held and the study needed a subject. Also, unlike most private patients, most clinic patients could not answer the question of why they had been asked to participate in the research. There were indications that the sole reason, in many cases, was the need for subjects. Most of the *unaware* subjects who were having elective (rather than medically required) inductions were patients of the house staff.

2. There are at least five different types of research subjects, based upon the reasons why subjects take part in research. The reasons for participation of only two of these types can be called reasons for *volunteering*. These are benefiting subjects, who participate for reasons of personal benefit (medical or convenience), and committed subjects, who volunteer out of a desire to help advance medical science.

Indifferent subjects give no reasons for participation and apparently acquiesce simply because a doctor asks them to do so. These subjects may not be aware that a choice is involved. Two categories of subjects most clearly do not consent—unwilling subjects, and those who are not aware that they are involved in research, unaware subjects.

3. Many factors can be involved in subjects' participation decisions. The importance or power of a number of decision factors was analyzed in Chapter Seven, and a number of hypotheses were offered as to how the importance of the various factors may vary from study to study. The appropriateness of factors considered by a subject in any particular study can be used as an indicator of valid consent. For example, in a risky study subjects should give thought to the question of risk. In a study of no benefit to subjects, subjects should indicate that altruistic reasons are important to their participation. The reasons given for participation can provide evidence of the validity of the consent process in a study.

4. A subject's signature on a consent form is no assurance that the subject has given informed consent. The most striking evidence of this was that almost 40 percent of the labor-induction subjects were unaware that research was involved in their inductions at the time they began receiving the drug. There were further indications of a lack of genuine informed consent.

Many subjects did not understand various aspects of the study, most gave no evidence of having given serious thought to a decision to participate, a few reported that they had felt pressured to participate, and many exhibited a lack of understanding of the decision-making aspects of the subject role.

Verbal acceptance by researchers of the idea of the subject's right to informed consent is quite different from their *determination to see that valid consent takes place.* The former, at minimum, may result in a signed consent form and the following of procedural requirements for the conduct of research. The latter would be reflected in such things as *personally* seeing that informed consent takes place rather than delegating the task, avoiding the use of euphemisms that fail to convey the desired information to prospective subjects, and, most importantly, seeing that an *oral* understanding is reached on key elements *in addition to* getting a signature on a piece of paper that describes those elements. For this, commitment to informed consent is necessary. Such a commitment probably cannot be assured solely through socialization in medical school and exposure to discussions of ethical issues. Nor do present procedural requirements provide sufficient stimulus.

5.   Many factors of greater or lesser importance interfere with a valid informed consent process. Included are factors that act to interfere with the subjects' freedom to refuse to participate, factors that result in the generally low level of understanding upon which many participation "decisions" are based, and the factor of general unpreparedness for the expectations of the role of research subject, particularly the requirement that a subject look out for his own interests.

There is no reason to think that the consent difficulties uncovered in this study are peculiar to a particular institution or to particular researchers. Rather we should look to the way in which research involving patients is generally conducted, and to the procedures that have been set forth to protect the rights of subjects.

6.   Some of the findings contribute toward an evaluation of DHEW's peer review requirements for the regulation of the conduct of human experimentation in the United States. Data on one peer review committee show that such committees can have an important impact on projects submitted to them (see Chapter Three). The Eastern University Clinical Research Committee commonly recommended ways to reduce the risk of projects and often required that consent forms be modified and clarified. On this level, my study provides support for a belief in the efficacy of such peer review procedures. (This is not to suggest that the CRC was doing the most effective job possible in this regard. To address the important question of how such things as the composition of a peer review committee and the types of procedures it follows affect its functioning, one would need

systematic comparative data on a number of different committees, along with a careful and detailed assessment of their effectiveness. The Barber group's study is a useful start in that direction.)[1]

It is one thing to say that a review committee has an impact on many proposed projects; it is quite another to say that such a committee has an impact on the actual conduct of research in an institution. If a committee does not use any regular monitoring system, it has no way of knowing whether projects that have never been approved are being conducted, whether approved projects are actually conducted according to the understanding between the investigator and the committee, and whether committee-approved procedures for securing the informed consent of subjects are actually effective for that purpose. My finding that informed consent often did not take place in a project that was approved by such a committee and that operated in accordance with the committee's stipulations leads to only one conclusion. The present policy of primary reliance on prior review is not adequate to assure that the actual conduct of research is in accordance with present ethical standards.

IMPLICATIONS OF THIS RESEARCH

The findings of this study, particularly those regarding informed consent, have a number of implications for subjects, for researchers, for the integrity of the research process, for the sociological problem of social control in professions, and for policy regulating the conduct of human experimentation.

Consent inadequacies have at least two consequences for human subjects. First, subjects are deprived of human rights about which there is widespread agreement. Beecher put it simply: "No man has the privilege of choosing participants for a risky procedure without the knowledge and agreement of the subject."[2] The first implication of this study, then, pertains to ethics: research is being done that violates fundamental ethical standards.

Inadequacies in the consent process have a second, less obvious consequence for subjects. This is illustrated by a subject who described her reactions to learning gradually about the research after she began labor:

R. Well, really the nurse and you [told me most about the research]. When I started talking to her about it . . . well it was after I talked to you actually. *That's* when I started asking her more. I was just asking her questions in general about being induced, you know, not knowing what was really going on. And then after talking with you I started asking a few more questions, but it didn't alarm me except it might have interested me more all of a sudden. I wasn't fearful at all. I thought it was kind of exciting, you know. (#36, white, private)

Lack of awareness, or poor understanding of research in which they are participants, deprives subjects of an experience that many might find rewarding.

The ethical problems raised by the use of subjects who have not given informed consent also threaten the integrity of the research process. This has been analyzed at length elsewhere, but the point is well stated by Paul Ramsey:

> Thus consent lies at the heart of medical care as a joint adventure between patient and doctor. It lies at the heart of man's continuing search for clues to all man's diseases as a great human adventure that is carried forward jointly by the investigator and his subjects. Stripped of the requirement of a reasonably free and an adequately informed consent, experimentation and medicine itself would speedily become inhumane.[3]

The consent inadequacies I have described also have implications for researchers. Since uninformed subjects are not likely to refuse or to ask difficult questions, a casual attitude toward informed consent may simplify the investigator's work in the short run. But it may prove to have long run effects that run counter to the interests of researchers.

On an immediate, personal level, consent inadequacies are potentially a source of serious legal difficulties. For one thing, informed consent provides the researcher with a defense to a battery charge. The law, in the words of Professor Freund, "is protective of human integrity and life. An offensive touching or invasion of the body, if not consented to, is a trespass against the person, a battery, redressable in an action for damages."[4] Furthermore, comments of several subjects in the present study suggest that the likelihood of a subject bringing such action is increased when a subject feels she has been misled or poorly informed. This was the source of genuine anger on the part of several subjects, and is evident in comments containing the hint of a threat against the investigators:

R. I know if, God forbid, something ever happened to this baby, and he came out and this and that was wrong with him. Of course, you get a lawyer and they would say, "Well, he was involved in an experiment. This drug is not proven yet." The hospital would be in for a lot of serious problems . . . They should have a form that says, you know,

"You hereby consent to involve yourself in an experimental drug that has been used successfully but is not yet proven." (#29, white, private)

R. I know, myself, God forbid, if something was wrong with the baby, which it's not, but if there were even the slightest thing wrong with her, even being a rational person and knowing that this could be caused by a physical thing other than this, I would have a tendency to doubt our decision, you know, and I think I would blame it on them [the researchers]. Which maybe isn't too rational, but you . . . because you're sort of forced into it. You know, you would say, "Well, gee, if I didn't do this or if you didn't force me, maybe this wouldn't have happened," though you realize that it's not from that. I think they could leave themselves wide open for a suit or something. (#24, white, private)

These comments from nonconsenting subjects—the first from an unaware subject, the second from one of the unwilling subjects—illustrate the increased legal danger faced by researchers when subjects can argue that their participation was not voluntary or informed. Almost all expressions of anger were centered around things subjects learned after the fact or things done that were at variance with subjects' prior understandings. Such misunderstandings may provide both the motivation and the legal basis for legal difficulties between investigators and subjects. That this is a consequence of inadequate consent procedures must be recognized.

The second consequence to researchers of consent inadequacies, although less direct and immediate, is perhaps of more long-term importance. Research that violates our ethical sensibilities may eventually poison the atmosphere in which clinical research is done and make successful solicitation of future subjects more problematic. There is good reason to believe that medical research is now well regarded by the general public, but it should not be assumed that this good will cannot be lost. Hans Jonas makes this point:

> in short, society cannot afford the absence among its members of *virtue* with its readiness to sacrifice beyond defined duty. Since its presence—that is to say, that of personal idealism—is a matter of grace and not a decree, we have the paradox that society depends for its existence on intangibles of nothing less than a religious order, for which it can hope, but which it cannot enforce. All the more must it protect this most precious capital from abuse.[5]

There is no reason why participation in research should be a negative experience.[6] On the contrary, acting as a research subject seems to have the potential of making enthusiasts out of some subjects—it can be an interesting, even exciting, experience. It also provides investigators with excellent opportunities to educate members of the public, which ultimately supports most research. However, if subjects feel that they have been taken advantage of by being exposed to risks and discomfort without giving informed consent, the experience of participating in research can create hostility toward researchers and antipathy toward research in general. One result can be pressure on government to tighten the rules under which experimentation is conducted. Though it would doubtless be resisted and resented, such action could well be in the interests of clinical investigators, because the long run effect of unethical research could be the destruction of an atmosphere of good will under which people are generally willing to help if asked. Quoting Beecher again, "society will not long tolerate the investigator's domination of another, with the possible expenditure of his subject's health or life. Studies that do not have at least the tacit support of the public will not flourish."[7]

A Note on the Use of Ward Patients as Research Subjects. In the existing American health care system, medical institutions such as hospitals commonly make a basic distinction between private patients and clinic or ward patients. This distinction is of course closely associated with such status variables as income and education, as seen in my study. Sociological studies have repeatedly shown that status differences are associated with a number of consequences in various settings. The overwhelming conclusion has been that patients of low social status are at a distinct disadvantage in our health (as well as other) institutions.[8]

One of the profound ethical and legal concerns that has arisen in human experimentation in recent years pertains to the suspected, but poorly documented, differential use as research subjects of clinic or ward patients, who tend to have relatively little education, income, and power. For example, Paul Freund said a few years ago:

> the concept of participation in decision-making may point up certain weaknesses in the concept of the constituency of patient-subjects. If it were the fact that patients on the wards were more freely used, or involved, in experimentation than those on private floors, some explanation would be called for . . .[9]

Others have suggested that if ward or clinic patients are, in fact, more likely than private patients to be used as research subjects, it is because these patients (like prisoners and students) are particularly convenient and accessible. However, data from the Barber group's study cast doubt on the adequacy of this explanation. Barber et al., using reports from clinical investigators, found that studies involving the highest levels of risks relative to benefit were the most likely to use ward patients as subjects.[10] This pattern of unequal distribution of risks and benefits cannot be explained by convenience and accessibility. My own study suggests another, more disturbing interpretation of the patterns of usage of ward or clinic patients as experimental subjects. This interpretation is based on what seems to be a reasonable assumption that researchers doing studies that have an unfavorable (for subjects) risk/benefit ratio would have the most difficulty in recruiting as subjects people who truly understand the risks and benefits and who give informed consent. Henry Beecher's famous article on apparently unethical published research studies[11] was based on the related notion that there are levels of risk that will not *knowingly* be assumed by ordinary individuals.

Beecher's method of examining published research reports did not illuminate how such individuals could become research subjects without realizing it. But my data simultaneously shed light on the way subjects can unknowingly become involved in research and on the patterns of research use of ward patients found by Barber et al. Consider these two findings. Research with unfavorable risk/benefit ratios is most likely to involve ward patients (Barber et al.), and ward patients are the most likely to become *unknowing* research subjects (my study). This suggests that research with unfavorable risk/benefit ratios is most likely to involve unknowing subjects, as Beecher assumed.

Several of the barriers to informed consent described in this study apply with particular force to ward or clinic patients, explaining why informed consent is more difficult to achieve with such subjects, as well as why it is easier for investigators to use such individuals as subjects without their knowledge. Recall that the greater the dissimilarity between investigator and subject in terms of such factors as education and race, the less likely was a subject to possess the basic knowledge that she was a research subject in the labor-induction study. Not only were these factors related to the acquiescence phenomenon, but subjects with low levels of education were most likely to exhibit the lack of sophistication about research that was reflected in the confusion between subject role expectations and patient role expectations, one barrier to consent.

In addition to the relative lack of both power and medical sophistication among ward patients, these patients are at an additional disadvantage because "their" physicians on the house staff are constrained to some extent to act as agents of medical school faculty members in locating suitable subjects for research. This finding has also been described in other settings by other investigators.[12] While there will certainly be individual variation among residents in enactment of this aspect of their role, they are nevertheless to an important extent dependent upon faculty members for assistance (consultations) while they are residents, and later for recommendations and sponsorship when they are ready to enter their postresidency careers, particularly careers in academic medicine.

The state of affairs in which individuals with whom informed consent is most difficult to achieve (and most easy to evade) are used as subjects in high risk/low benefit research (in which the self-protection functions of informed consent are most relevant) differs markedly from the ideal approach envisaged a few years ago by the philosopher Hans Jonas:

> one should look for subjects where a maximum of identification [with the purpose of the research], understanding, and spontaneity can be expected—that is, among the most highly motivated, the most highly educated, and the least "captive" members of the community. From this naturally scarce resource, a descending order of permissibility leads to greater abundance and ease of supply, whose use should become proportionately more hesitant as the exculpating criteria are relaxed. An inversion of normal "market" behavior is demanded here— namely, to accept the lowest quotation last (and excused only by the greatest pressure of need), to pay the highest price first.[13]

Such a reversal of market behavior—seeking highly educated subjects for research that has relatively unfavorable risk/benefit ratios—would also be a reversal of present practices as indicated by the Barber group's work and by my own study. The most efficient way of producing such a state of affairs is to enact procedures that would help assure that *genuine* informed consent is a primary goal for clinical investigators.

Social Control Implications. Broadly speaking, this study has two important implications for the principle of informed consent. First, the presence of some well-informed volunteers in both studies shows that informed consent is not an unrealistic goal, as has sometimes been suggested. Second, the presence of many uninformed and poorly informed subjects demonstrates that informed consent is not always an easy goal to achieve (which no one has suggested). It is certainly more complex than getting a subject to sign a consent form.

The securing of genuine informed consent from research subjects clearly requires sincere effort by investigators. Of course, the investigator must present to prospective subjects the facts regarding risks, benefits, purpose, alternatives, and so forth, as DHEW policy[14] now specifies. This task should not be delegated, for reasons described in Chapter Eight. Furthermore, the investigator must also be prepared to acquaint subjects with certain key aspects of the subject role—specifically, that the subject is being asked to volunteer for something that is not required, that he does not have to volunteer just because a doctor asks him to do so, that he should feel free to refuse and not be concerned about reprisals, that it is appropriate to ask any questions he may have, and that he may withdraw at any time. Finally, when everything has been explained, the investigator (or a third party) must question the subject to assure that communication has taken place and that the subject understands the information.

This study shows without question that informed consent is not achieved simply by making information available to subjects with no further explanation or discussion. Consent forms play a useful role in the process of getting informed consent from subjects.[15] But researchers must understand that a written consent form does not in and of itself constitute an adequate means of informing subjects, and that it should not be the only information given to subjects. Consent forms should provide a written statement of an understanding reached between an investigator and prospective subject prior to the subject's signing of the form. It should be less of a device for communicating information than a means for providing assurance to subjects that the investigator has verbally covered all points thought to be necessary by a peer review committee.

Assuring that investigators will seriously strive to secure the informed consent of subjects is an interesting and somewhat difficult social control problem. Getting informed consent from subjects not only requires effort; it also means spending time for which the investigator is not directly rewarded, time that involves an intangible task that is incidental to his primary goal.

As one examines the literature on human experimentation to see how the problems of ethics in research and the means of assuring ethical performance are dealt with, certain emphases are readily apparent. Many thoughtful and sensitive statements about the practices that *should* occur in clinical investigation can be found. The following statements by Dr. De Bakey and Dr. Beecher are typical:

> The investigator must never permit his zeal for research or his self-interest to blunt his reverence for human life and the right of self-determination. . . . It is incumbent on every member of a research team and on the administrative personnel of related medical and scientific institutions, as well as related lay and governmental agencies, to maintain the highest standards of research and to prevent breaches of medical ethics by careful evaluation of proposed investigative procedures.[16]

the patient's welfare must not take second place to education and the advancement of knowledge. The doctor-investigator cannot be any more neglectful of the interest of a group of individuals under his responsibility in the laboratory, for the sake of science, than he is of one patient in his consulting room who comes for therapy.[17]

The many statements echoing these goals no doubt serve useful functions in affecting the moral climate in which research is done and in sensitizing readers to the various issues involved.

In comparison, relatively little serious consideration has been given to mechanisms or procedures that might help assure that the ideals are achieved.* Most suggestions that are offered, such as the proposal to increase attention to ethical issues in medical education, are extremely general. And one repeatedly encounters variations of the argument that the ideals cannot be achieved by a system of regulation but must be left to the moral integrity of the individual and his peers. For example, Dr. DeBakey argues in the article quoted above that "ethical decisions in medical science must depend finally on the wisdom, integrity, and self-imposed restraints of the scientist and his peers."[18] Dr. Beecher takes a similar position, saying that "security rests with the *responsible* investigator, who will refer decisions to his peers."[19] The social control problem, of course, is how to assure that those ethical decisions will be made properly or referred to peers as they should be. Nor does offering this concern imply that investigators lack moral integrity. One only has to recognize that in many situations the ethical requirements are ambiguous, that various situational pressures impinge on the investigator, and that the investigator has strong scientific and career interests that hardly make him a disinterested decision-maker.

One reason for the preponderance of attention to ideals as compared to mechanisms for achieving them in the literature is that little data have been available on actual practices. This study is, of course, directed at illuminating the practices that take place in human experimentation, and it has some obvious implications for the general problem of the social control of the behavior of professionals, a matter that is of sociological and of policy interest.

A central characteristic that distinguishes the professions from other occupations is the extent to which professional social control is based on self-

---

* DeBakey's statement does mention a mechanism—evaluation of *proposed* procedures. However, this is suggested as a way of preventing breeches of medical ethics, and since the most important breaches occur after the proposal stage of research, the mechanism (which already existed at the time he wrote) is hardly to the point, even though it can have an important role in affecting the kind of research that is done.

regulation. This autonomy is generally based on three claims: that the knowledge needed to evaluate the performance of the professional is beyond that possessed by laymen, that professionals are responsible and so may be trusted to work conscientiously without supervision, and that the profession itself will undertake regulatory action should it be required.[20] Elsewhere Freidson has pointed out that the evidence suggests that visibility of performance is the key to social control of professionals.[21] One reason why medical practice itself has traditionally been so difficult to regulate is because the performance of the physician—particularly the solo practitioner who has long dominated the organization of the American health care system—is visible only to individual patients.

The only visible aspect of the ethical performance of the clinical investigator is ordinarily the consent form, which, as the data on the labor-induction subjects demonstrates, can be signed without informed consent taking place. (The technical aspects of the research are made visible to some extent by the fact that the research results will have to withstand professional scrutiny in the scientific literature. No such scrutiny of the ethical performance of the investigator is at present part of the structure of the conduct of the research, although the suggestion that professional journals review that aspect before accepting papers for publication[22] is a gesture in that direction.) I suspect that if the data existed one would find that the less visible a piece of research—that is, the more it resembles ordinary diagnosis or therapy or the greater the extent to which the researcher works alone—the less likely to be followed are the basic procedural requirements of submission to peer review and use of consent forms.

While the importance of visibility may seem apparent, the present regulation of the conduct of human experimentation relies almost entirely on the socialization of investigators in their training and on prior review of proposed research. As pointed out in Chapter Three, peer review committees do not seem anxious to assume the role of policeman, perhaps because such a role might imply that their colleagues, and therefore they themselves, cannot be trusted to behave correctly in the absence of a detection mechanism. That committee members, most of whom are physicians, are reluctant to assume such a role should probably not be surprising. After all, the notion that professionals do not need to be monitored underlies the way our society has chosen to regulate the behavior of professionals. Historically in the United States, the main approach to regulating professionals and assuring that they are practicing in a proper fashion has been through procedures applied before the professional begins practice. The major mechanism is the licensing procedure, which is supposed to weed out people of inadequate competence. Once licensed, the practitioner's competence is never again examined, even if he practices for

40 or more years. Licensing agencies usually reenter the picture only if the professional gets into legal difficulties.[23]

Similarly, the review procedure is supposed to weed out ethically unacceptable projects and to set the basic ground rules to which the investigator is supposed to conform. Once that is done, the review committee's role virtually ends, although investigators are instructed to inform the committee of changes in their projects. This is why I characterize the present regulation of human experimentation as based almost entirely on prior regulation.

I should also like to offer a few comments about the socialization of investigators, upon which present policy de facto relies. It is true that medical students are increasingly being exposed to ethical issues in medicine, including clinical investigation, and this is all to the good. However, faith that better ethical training for investigators will by itself solve the problems in the ethical conduct of research needs to be strongly tempered.

First, there is no evidence that exposure to ethical issues in the training of the investigator is associated with eventual behavior differences. Barber et al. found that such training in and of itself was not even associated with *expressed* ethical standards, except in the presence of such structural factors as interaction patterns and authority structures.[24] Second, ethical training received years before may fade in the presence of situational pressures that make the cutting of ethical corners expedient.

There are certainly reasons to view ethical training in medical education as desirable. Among other things, it can to some extent countervail some of the authoritarian ways of dealing with problems that are transmitted in medical education. That is, there are emphases in the training of physicians that may interfere with the type of sharing of decisions that is implied by the concept of informed consent. Sociological studies of medical education have found, for example, that a major emphasis in the clinical years is the exercise of medical responsibility. The physician-in-training becomes accustomed to holding the patient's fate in his hands.[25] While this is necessary, there is danger here, as Jay Katz noted in his article on the education of the physician-investigator:

> Traditionally the concept of medical responsibility has been defined as responsibility for the patient's well-being. While such a definition could encompass, within the context of a medical relationship, concern for the patient's functioning—physical, psychological, social, economic, spiritual—it is often limited to physical aspects. In order to exercise this more limited responsibility, patients must be carefully diagnosed, given the best

treatment for their condition, and not be abandoned. Many students learn well to fulfill these obligations. But there are other aspects to medical responsibility, and the controversy about what to disclose to patient-subjects in investigative settings has put one of them into sharper perspective—namely, the dialogue that should be pursued with the patient about treatment or no treatment or available alternative treatments in light of the risks, benefits, and prognosis as well as the totality of the patient's life situation. Put another way, so long as medical responsibility primarily addressed itself to dispensing physical benefits, it was easier to view the physician as the sole decision-maker. Once physical benefits are placed in the web of the patient's total situation, the patient may have to be given a greater role in the decision-making process.[26]

An excellent example of how an investigator's willingness to assume responsibility can interfere with a genuine consent process is cited by Beecher. In an article in *Anesthesiology*, distinguished investigator-authors stated that because they believed that it was impossible to transmit to subjects the information necessary to informed consent, they instead "accepted the role of guarantor of the patient's rights and safety."[27] Beecher offers a thorough critique of this approach, noting among other things that

an adoption of the paternalistic view recommended really leaves all decision-making to the investigator; what should be a joint enterprise between subject and investigator becomes a monopoly of the investigator, who is thus unhampered by personal discussion with the subject of the latter's wishes and interests. There would be no limitations . . . if the policy stated here were to be generally adopted.[28]

The labor-induction study was carried out by an investigator who expressed considerable awareness of ethical issues and who followed current procedural requirements for assuring that the research was ethically sound. Nevertheless, it suffered from consent problems, and thus suggests that reliance solely upon investigator ethicality (a product of socialization) and prior approval of projects by a review committee is not sufficient. Before offering suggestions for modification of present policy, I would like to consider briefly an explanation of why existing social control measures do not suffice.

The answer lies, I believe, in the role expectations and career interests of investigators* and the situational pressures they face. Professional reputa-

* Here I am using the term "investigator" generically, and do not aim my remarks specifically at the investigators whose subjects I interviewed. I have no way of knowing whether this analysis applies to them.

tions and positions, particularly at certain career stages, depend primarily on publishing research results. More than intelligence, skill, and imagination are required to conduct research. There are many practical problems as well. Funds must be sought to support the research. Because of the need to bring various kinds of expertise to bear on different aspects of the research, collaboration may be necessary, bringing with it another set of problems. Access must be gained to facilities—hospital beds for research purposes may be allocated by a special committee, for example. Then, it is necessary to secure approval of the peer review committee. The conduct of the research may involve the investigator in the management and coordination of a group of assistants and technicians, and he must manage his other responsibilities (additional research projects, teaching, patient care, committee work, and so forth) at the same time. And, of course, he must locate subjects.

Research involves substantial rewards in prestige, position, and satisfaction for the investigator, and involves a great many practical problems as well. Attempts to reduce these day-to-day problems are to be expected, particularly when their only cost is intangible and diffuse. In addition, the high value placed on "advancing medical knowledge" makes convenient the belief that a higher goal is being pursued. And this belief can come to excuse liberties taken with ethical niceties and may salve the conscience.

So it should not surprise us if there exists a pattern of approaching individuals from the least educated and most powerless segments of society for research that carries relatively high risk in proportion to the benefits to subjects. Nor should we be surprised when an investigator delegates responsibility for getting subjects' consent; he delegates as many "routine" tasks as he can. Nor at the willingness of some investigators to evade the peer review procedure altogether or to conduct their research contrary to the manner approved by the committee. Nor if the formal aspects of consent are allowed to substitute for its substance. Above all, we should not be surprised by any of these occurrences when investigators can have a high degree of confidence that their conduct will never be subject to review.

To return again to the regulation of the ordinary practice of medicine, it is generally agreed that the examination and licensing procedure is a useful device for helping assure that beginning practitioners meet certain minimum standards. However, it is becoming increasingly obvious that primary reliance on prior means of social control of an entire profession is naive at best. At worst, it is a self-serving device for maintaining a fiction that the profession is a responsible body that regulates itself for the public's protection. Critics have pointed out that the lack of periodic review of credentials and the infrequency of disciplinary actions against practitioners belie claims that licensing procedures insure the quality of professional practice, and a few states are beginning to require the periodic reexamination of physicians. Furthermore, recent developments in computer technology, the institutionalization of health care, and medicine's success in reaching some standards of treatment upon which there is some agreement have made the monitoring of physicians' behavior and comparing their practices against standards of good medical practice increasingly feasible.[29] If actual care rendered by physicians could be judged against accepted standards, poor practices would be made visible, and appropriate actions could be taken. A priori, it would seem likely that a practitioner's awareness that his work is subject to review would be an effective spur for him to stay abreast of developments in his field.

There seems to be no necessary reason why formal social control of human experimentation should rely primarily upon prior committee review. My own data show that while this procedure can have an important impact on proposed research, prior review is not effective in assuring ethical behavior in clinical investigation, particularly with regard to informed consent. If there exists a true commitment to assuring that research is conducted in an ethical fashion, a mechanism must be created that will *detect* unethical practices and make them visible. If investigators are aware that their dealings with subjects will be scrutinized, one can expect them to avoid careless or devious methods of seeking consent. The standards against which an investigator's ethical performance should be judged may not pose a serious problem. It is the peer review committee's job to decide how the abstract general ethical principles are to be applied in concrete situations. It is their job to decide whether written consent is necessary, what risks subjects should be apprised of, and so forth.

The needed visibility of ethical performance could result from the operation of a regular monitoring procedure in which someone, probably a representative of the institutional review committee, determines whether subjects knew they were in research, whether they understood the risks, benefits, and alternatives, and whether they felt free to refuse to participate. This information would have to come from interviews with *subjects,* not from data furnished by investigators.

My experience shows that it may not be difficult to learn the extent of subjects' knowledge about these matters. I am not proposing that such an interview take place before subjects' participation in research actually begins for several reasons. The mechanics of arranging interviews between the time subjects give consent and the time their participation begins are forbidding. Such an arrangement would put the monitor in an awkward position and could make the researcher-subject relationship more difficult. Such a procedure is not necessary to achieve the goal of assuring that informed consent takes place. I am suggesting the less direct, but more efficient, procedure of interviewing randomly selected subjects* after they have participated in research. That way, the problems mentioned above would be avoided, and the monitor would not be put into the position of having responsibility for *informing* subjects. That, of course, is the investigator's responsibility. Relatively few subjects would need to be interviewed, which would minimize the administration and cost of the monitoring procedure.

In brief, an *institutionalized mechanism for detecting ethical evasions or sloppiness* must be established. If a pattern of participation based upon constraint, poor understanding, or misunderstanding were found among an investigator's subjects, a range of options could apply. At minimum, investigators could be advised how to avoid future deficiencies in securing the informed consent of subjects. Warnings could be issued. Willful or persistent violations of ethical standards would call for more serious steps, such as temporary or permanent suspension in funding or in access to facilities.

This monitoring procedure is not proposed as an alternative to the existing review procedure, but would supplement that valuable mechanism. The expert knowledge represented on a review committee is necessary for making the essential judgments about whether proposed research procedures minimize possible risks to subjects. A review committee composed of professional and lay members is uniquely suited to determining whether the remaining risks are justified by the scientific merits of the proposed research, a judgment about which an investigator might not be objective.

Institutional review committees must also play an important role in assessing whether proposed means of securing informed consent are adequate. In this area there are again good reasons why technical expertise (which is needed to assure that the form is technically accurate and complete) should be supplemented by lay points of view. Nonexperts can play an important role in assuring that consent forms are comprehensible and sufficiently noneuphemistic to get the necessary point across to prospective subjects that a *voluntary* decision is being requested for participation in medical *research*. A monitoring procedure that reveals what subjects do and do not understand about research could provide committees with essential feedback on whether the consent forms they approve provide subjects with the necessary information in a manner in which it can be understood.

This discussion of social control mechanisms has been confined to formal

---

* A useful procedural step would be a requirement that investigators furnish central registries at their institutions with the names of research subjects. It is presently difficult to determine how many patients at an institution are involved in research, who the patients are, and whether they are taking part in one or in several studies. A central registry would make the monitoring of the use of human subjects far more feasible.

procedures, which submit most readily to revision and amendment. However, the role of informal social control measures requires comment. One distinguished investigator has asserted that:

> In the control of individual behavior of physicians, social restraints have undoubtedly been more effective than the legal ones. Once a physician is licensed, his behavior in the most important areas has been influenced much more by his need and desire for the respect of his professional peers than by any legal constraints upon his actions. Aside from the fact that licensure is limited to individuals with a certain minimum educational achievement, the high general quality of medical care in the United States is due not to legal force, but rather to the intangible social forces that motivate individual behavior. It is intolerable to a physician to be considered a stupid, lazy or unethical person by his or her professional peers; and, fortunately for society, the profession of medicine attracts persons of such intellectual ability, because it offers opportunity both for intellectual and social satisfaction, that a relatively high standard of performance is set as the norm. If this were not so, no amount of legal machinery could enforce intelligent and ethical practice.[30]

While few sociologists would discount the social control role of such informal factors as approval of peers, it should be recognized that such controls are not sufficient. Work by Beecher, Pappworth, Barber's group, and myself suggests that a significant amount of ethically deficient research takes place,[31] even though the informal controls of peer approval or disapproval are presumably in operation. There are several reasons why such controls are not adequate.

For peer disapproval of one's conduct to have an effect, investigators would have to be quite familiar with each other's practices with regard to such matters as informing subjects. However, as I have pointed out, the interaction between researcher and subject is rarely highly visible. Thus, investigators may not know very much about what their colleagues are doing with regard to consent. The monitoring procedure proposed above might have an impact on this situation.

In addition, peer disapproval can be ignored or explained away. Also, the assertion that fear of offending peer standards will control individual behavior assumes a higher degree of consensus on standards than the Barber group's evidence shows to exist.[32] Work by Freidson and Rhea[33] and by the Barber group[34] indicates that physicians and investigators tend to work with individuals who share their professional and ethical standards, which suggests that one's contacts with peers who might disapprove of one's behavior may be limited by choice. Finally, the immediacy of the role and career pressures discussed earlier may be sufficient to override concerns about peer disapproval. For all of these reasons, informal control by peer approval or disapproval, while important, is hardly sufficient. This is a difficult social control mechanism to modify, except insofar as the procedural proposals I have offered will make investigators' practices vis-à-vis research subjects more visible.

It is apparent, then, that present methods of control over the conduct of clinical investigation in the United States are not adequate to assure that such research meets currently accepted ethical standards. My evidence suggests that prior review of proposed research by institutional review committees has been a useful step in protecting the rights and welfare of subjects, but that primary reliance on prior review as a means of influencing the behavior of researchers is not adequate. The performance of professionals in this important area cannot safely be left solely to such prior monitoring procedures, since there is enormous potential for the occurrence of unethical practices in the absence of visibility of actions by practitioners.

THE DISCREPANCY BETWEEN STANDARDS AND PRACTICES

This study was intended from its inception to focus on topics of sociological interest. Insofar as such issues as the social control of professionals, the nature of the doctor-patient relationship, and the social bases of the act of volunteering have been examined, it has retained that sociological focus. However, it is the *ethical* issues raised in human experimentation that are ultimately the most compelling. Although these issues have received much attention, precious little information on how actual practices compare with the basic ethical requirements has been available. This study has empirically examined some heretofore unexamined facets of the conduct of human experimentation. In this last section I want to consider briefly the questions raised by the discrepancies between our practices and our ideals, particularly with regard to the two major issues of risk/benefit ratio and informed consent.*

* A third ethical issue, which operates at quite a different level, should also be mentioned again—whether the risks and benefits of research are distributed within the population in a manner that will withstand scrutiny, that is, in a manner that does not offend our standards of equity. While no study of the epidemiology of research subjectdom has been done, the Barber group's study indicates that research in which risks to subjects are not balanced by benefits is most likely to use as subjects individuals from the least affluent and educated segments of American society. In addition, an ample body of literature shows that these same groups are least likely to receive good medical care, that is, to receive the benefits of past research. (This may not be true at the individual level, however. It may be that those who are in institutions in which medical research is done are the first to benefit from knowledge gained in earlier re-

Although difficult to state in operational terms, there is little dispute that the risks to subjects in a study should be outweighed by its potential benefits, either to subjects or to a body of knowledge. Whether a justifiable risk/benefit ratio exists in any particular study, however, is a matter about which reasonable people can differ. Nevertheless, a potentially effective mechanism—the institutional review committees—has been created to deal with the issue in actual cases. A broadly constituted committee is at least in the position to make such decisions. The concept seems to be appropriate. At the same time, Chapter Three shows that there is good reason to believe that most institutional review committees are inactive and ineffective. Useful research could further study the structural bases of the variations between institutional committees in how seriously they pursue their functions.

However, it is with informed consent that the most substantial discrepancy exists between what is supposed to occur and what actually takes place. Compared with the risk/benefit question, resolution of the informed consent issue in a routinized fashion in actual cases is considerably more difficult. The risk/benefit judgment can often be made only one time per study. That is, the review committee deals with the issue one time, before the start of a study, by deciding whether or not the study's benefits outweigh the risks that subjects will be asked to assume.[35] In contrast, the issue of informed consent applies to individual subjects, not to complete studies. Notwithstanding this fact, the existing review requirements attempt to handle the informed consent issue as if it too can be decided on a study-by-study basis, by making a single judgment before the research begins about whether the proposed means of seeking informed consent are adequate. While making a single determination that the informed consent issue is being dealt with adequately by an investigator is certainly convenient, my interviews with subjects show that even under favorable conditions a prior committee review has little bearing on whether eventual subjects' participation will be based on informed consent. Here there appears to be a discrepancy between the goal to be achieved—informed consent—and the procedure that is supposed to achieve it, prior committee review.

Finally, I wish to consider briefly the choice we face when we discover serious ethical shortcomings in an activity that is greatly valued and

---

search.) Responsibility for this risk/benefit pattern is difficult to fix, because it is a result of *many* investigators' selection of subjects. To the extent that the pattern of differential exposure to risks and benefits results from the organization and financing of health care in this country, procedural requirements are not a useful way of approaching the problem. To the extent that the pattern is based on the ease of evading informed consent requirements with subjects who have relatively little education and power, procedures that make informed consent a more *effective* requirement can be expected to alter the situation.

willingly supported by our society. If existing social control mechanisms do not assure that human experimentation is conducted in a way that does not violate our ethical standards, then we face three options.

We can acknowledge the existence of ethical shortcomings revealed by empirical work on the conduct of human experimentation and try to meet the problem. Out of the two major empirical efforts of recent years—the Barber group's work and this study—have come concrete suggestions for policy changes. My own major suggestion is recognition of the need to monitor the ethical performance of investigators as a regular procedure, and the creation of mechanisms to achieve this end. This suggestion is based on the argument that the lack of visibility of the consent situation is a major contributing factor in the lack of informed consent in research.

A second choice is to ignore the problem, to deny its existence. To do this, the empirical work that demonstrates the existing ethical shortcomings must either be disregarded or discredited.

The third, and I suspect most probable, reaction is to acknowledge the existence of ethical problems but to argue that the costs of correcting the problem are excessive. In this vein are assertions that any impediments to progress in combating cancer, heart disease, mental retardation, arthritis, and so on are against the public interest.

This takes us back to the point made early in Chapter One—the use of human subjects in research involves goal and value conflicts. These conflicts, which make the topic so fascinating and complex, operate on many levels.* Perhaps the generic conflict is between the scientist's desire to conduct research that will advance scientific knowledge and (presumably) eventually benefit mankind, and the need to uphold cultural conceptions of individual dignity and rights. However, the question of whether the regulation or monitoring of an activity such as human experimentation will unnecessarily hamper scientific advances needs some comment.

With regard to the assertion that procedures that aim to assure that our *existing* ethical principles are upheld are unnecessary impediments to medical progress, it needs to be recognized that the conflict is largely between ethics and scientific progress, not between procedures and scientific progress. There seems to me to be little question that the use of subjects *only with their informed consent* will be more costly in time and effort than the use of subjects without their informed consent. Seeking genuine

---

* Jay Katz, for example, has pointed out that human experimentation involves conflicts between our desire to expand knowledge and our fears of the unknown and desire to perpetuate the status quo, between the inevitability of injury to life and limb in all of our activities and the belief in the paramount value of every human life, between the need and wish to rely on the expertise of professionals and man's desire to control the decisions that affect his life. *Experimentation with Human Beings* (New York: Russell Sage, 1972), pp. 111–112.

consent will be costly because it requires time and effort and will result in a larger number of people refusing to be subjects. Yet, while I know of no one arguing against the general validity of the informed consent requirement, resistance to procedures to guarantee it is likely. However, if informed consent is indeed typical in an investigator's research, a monitoring procedure such as was suggested in the preceding section will in no way slow the progress of medical research, because such a procedure would enter the picture only following subjects' involvement in research. If informed consent is not taking place, however, a procedure that puts new pressure on investigators to secure informed consent may mean a change in the ease with which subjects are recruited. This change should be attributed to the upholding of existing standards, not to the procedure that is developed for that purpose.

The conflict is not only between ethical conduct and the widely supported goal of "medical progress," however. The conflict is also between ethics and the immediate career interests of investigators in an academic system that emphasizes research and publication. It is convenient to wrap those ambitions in the cloak of benefits to mankind, but the career interests themselves should not be overlooked. The Barber group found that career pressures had a measurable impact on the ethical standards of investigators.[36]

To the question of whether upholding ethical standards is worth some cost in the rapidity of medical progress, I would in conclusion offer the answer given a few years ago by Hans Jonas:

> Let us not forget that progress is an optional goal, not an unconditional commitment, and that its tempo in particular, compulsive as it may become, has nothing sacred about it. Let us also remember that a slower progress in the conquest of disease would not threaten society, grievous as it is to those who have to deplore that their particular disease be not yet conquered, but that society would indeed be threatened by the erosion of those moral values whose loss, probably caused by too ruthless a pursuit of scientific progress, would make its most dazzling triumphs not worth having.[37]

NOTES

1. See particularly Chapter Nine, "Social Control: The Structures, Processes, and Efficacy of Peer Group Review," in Bernard Barber et al., *Research on Human Subjects* (New York: Russell Sage, 1973).

2. Henry K. Beecher, *Research and the Individual: Human Studies* (Boston: Little, Brown, 1970), p. 24.

3. Paul Ramsey, *The Patient as Person—Explorations in Medical Ethics* (New Haven: Yale University Press, 1970), p. 11.

4. Paul A. Freund, "Ethical Problems in Human Experimentation," *New England Journal of Medicine,* 273 (1965), 687–692. Quoted in Beecher, *op. cit.,* p. 24.

5. Hans Jonas, "Philosophical Reflections on Experimenting with Human Subjects," *Daedalus,* 98 (Spring 1969), 229.

6. In fact, altruistic motivations are rewarded by such acts of volunteering. See, for example, Richard M. Titmuss, *The Gift Relationship: From Human Blood to Social Policy* (New York: Pantheon, 1971).

7. Beecher, op. cit., p. 24.

8. See, for example, A. B. Hollingshead and F. C. Redlich, *Social Class and Mental Illness* (New York: Wiley, 1958); David Sudnow, *Passing On: The Social Organization of Dying,* (Englewood Cliffs, N.J.: Prentice-Hall, 1967); Raymond S. Duff and A. B. Hollingshead, *Sickness and Society* (New York: Harper & Row, 1968); Julius A. Roth, "Some Contingencies of the Moral Evaluation and Control of Clientele: The Case of the Hospital Emergency Room," *American Journal of Sociology,* 77 (1972), 839–856.

9. Paul A. Freund, "Legal Frameworks for Human Experimentation," *Daedalus,* 98 (Spring 1968), 318.

10. Barber et al., op. cit., pp. 53–57.

11. "Ethics and Clinical Research," *New England Journal of Medicine,* 274 (1966), 1354–1360.

12. See Stephen J. Miller, *Prescription for Leadership: Training for the Medical Elite* (Chicago: Aldine, 1970), pp. 145–154. See also Barber et al., op. cit., pp. 104–107.

13. Jonas, op. cit., p. 235.

14. *The Institutional Guide to DHEW Policy on Protection of Human Subjects.* DHEW Publication No. (NIH) 72-102.

15. To my knowledge only one little-known article has presented any data on the impact of the introduction of written consent forms into a research project: Audrey T. McCollum and A. Herbert Schwartz, "Pediatric Research Hospitalization: Its Meaning to Parents," *Pediatric Research,* 3 (1969), 199–204. McCollum and Schwartz conducted a series of interviews with parents of children being hospitalized in a pediatric research center. During this series of interviews, which were directed at determining parental understanding of the research nature of their children's hospitalization, the PHS peer review requirements took effect (October, 1966), and the investigators began to obtain written consent prior to children's admission to the hospital. McCollum and Schwartz found that "prior to the existence of this policy [mandatory protocol review prior to admission and written consent forms], 69% of the mothers believed the purpose of the hospitalization to be entirely diagnostic or therapeutic. Subsequently, only 19% presented this view" (p. 202). Surprisingly, even with this finding McCollum and Schwartz imply that the lack of informed consent was the *parents'* fault, due to their utilization of "denial and repression in blocking these anxiety-producing communications" (p. 199). Yet their own data show that parents' awareness of the research depended upon which of the eight investigators "informed" them. None of the parents who dealt with one of the investigators was aware of the research, unlike *all* of the parents who dealt with another one. Such variation among investigators hardly suggests that the uninformed parents were responsible for the situation.

16. Michael E. DeBakey, "Medical Research and the Golden Rule," *Journal of the American Medical Association,* 203 (19 February 1968), 133–134.

17. Beecher, op. cit., p. 90.

18. DeBakey, op. cit., p. 134.

19. Beecher, op. cit., p. 23.

20. Eliot Freidson, *The Profession of Medicine* (New York: Dodd, Mead, 1970), p. 137.

21. Eliot Freidson, *Professional Dominance: The Social Structure of Medical Care* (New York: Atherton, 1970), p. 90.

22. Henry Beecher is one who has suggested this. See *Research and the Individual,* pp. 31–32 and 290–291.

23. Robert C. Derbyshire, *Medical Licensure and Discipline in the United States* (Baltimore: Johns Hopkins, 1969), particularly Chapter Six.

24. Barber et al., op. cit., p. 94.

25. Howard S. Becker, Blanche Geer, Everett C. Hughes, and Anselm L. Strauss, *Boys in White: Student Culture in Medical School* (Chicago: University of Chicago Press, 1961), pp. 224–231.

26. Jay Katz, "The Education of the Physician-Investigator," *Daedalus,* 98 (Spring 1969), 485.

27. G. Long, R. D. Dripps, and H. L. Price, "Measurement of Anti-Arrhythmic Potency of Drugs in Man: Effects of Dehydrobenzperidol," *Anesthesiology,* 28 (1967), 318–323. Beecher's discussion is in *Research and the Individual,* pp. 27–29.

28. Beecher, op. cit., p. 29.

29. These factors are examined by Laurence R. Tancredi and John Woods, "The Social Control of Medical Practice," *Milbank Memorial Fund Quarterly,* 50 (1972), 99–125.

30. Maurice B. Visscher, "The Two Sides of the Coin in the Regulation of Experimental Medicine," *Annals of the New York Academy of Science,* 169 (January 1970), 321.

31. I am referring to Beecher's article, "Ethics and Clinical Research," *New England Journal of Medicine,* 274 (1966), 1354–1360, and M. H. Pappworth's book, *Human Guinea Pigs* (Boston: Beacon, 1968). The Barber group's book has been cited numerous times.

32. *Research on Human Subjects,* Chapter Three.

33. Eliot Freidson and Buford Rhea, "Processes of Control in a Company of Equals," *Social Problems,* 2 (1963), 119–131.

34. *Research on Human Subjects,* Chapter Seven.

35. However, it is obvious that in a study using a heterogeneous sample the risk/benefit ratio may vary from subject to subject. Some may be more likely to benefit from the research, or it might be more risky for certain types of subjects. The extent to which review committee actions reflect recognition of this fact is not known.

36. *Research on Human Subjects,* Chapters Four and Five.

37. Jonas, op. cit., p. 245.

CONSENT FORM:
LABOR-INDUCTION STUDY

Patient Consent Form for Participation in A Clinical Investigation Project

"Eastern" University School of Medicine

Description of Project:

Your physician has decided to start you in labor. This is usually done by giving a drug called pitocin. Recently, two new drugs called (X) and (Y) have also been shown to efficiently and safely start labor. This study will compare the three drugs, therefore, you will receive one of the three. (X) and (Y) are experimental drugs which will be given intravenously, as is pitocin. The usage of (X) and (Y) is limited in this country. Although adverse effects are possible with any new drug, none have been noted with (X) or (Y). It is routine on our service for patients being induced in labor to have electronic monitoring of the baby's heart rate and the uterine contractions for safety purposes—this will be done after the procedure is fully explained to you.

Authorization: I have read the above and agree to participation in the project described above. Its general purposes, potential benefits, and possible hazards and inconveniences have been explained to my satisfaction.

. . . .
Signature

. . . .
Date

. . . .
(Physician)

SUBJECT QUESTIONNAIRE:
CLINICAL INVESTIGATION STUDY*

1. Name of Project _____

2. Name of Respondent _____

3. Date _____

4. Place of Interview _____

5. Respondent's Address _____

    _____ Local (city)
    _____ Local (suburb)
    _____ In-state
    _____ Other

6. Respondent's Sex

    _____ Male
    _____ Female

7. Respondent's Race or Ethnic Group

    _____ White
    _____ Black, other than Spanish-speaking

* Items are presented as used in the labor-induction study—that is, several items not used with starvation-abortion subjects are included. When the interview schedule was prepared, the projects in which subjects would be interviewed had not been identified. Hence, questions specific to the labor-induction study in particular were added at the last minute. Also, since some of the original research questions concerned differences between those who volunteer and those who refuse, and none of the latter were encountered, some items that were included in the schedule were not included in the analysis presented in this book. Throughout, items presented to subjects are capitalized. Where response categories are capitalized, they were presented to subjects as alternatives.

_____ Spanish-speaking
_____ Other

8. COULD WE HAVE A LITTLE INFORMATION ON YOUR
   HOUSEHOLD? WHO IS THE HEAD OF THE HOUSEHOLD? [At
   this point a chart (not reproduced here) was completed on which was included the name of each family member, relationship to the head of the
   household (for example, spouse, parent), age, sex, marital status, education,
   and occupation. These items were coded as follows:]

   a. Head of Household

      _____ Respondent
      _____ Spouse
      _____ Parent
      _____ Other relative
      _____ Other

   b. Respondent's Marital Status

      _____ Never married
      _____ Married
      _____ Separated
      _____ Divorced
      _____ Widowed

   c. Respondent's Age (not recoded)

   d. Number in Household (coded one to eight or more)

   e. Number Dependent upon Respondent (and Spouse) for Support (coded
      one to eight or more)

   f. Respondent's Education

      _____ Graduate or professional training
      _____ College degree
      _____ Some college
      _____ High school degree
      _____ Some high school (10th or 11th grade completed)
      _____ Junior high school (grade 7–9 completed)
      _____ Less than 7 years of school

   g. Respondent's Occupation (categories from Hollingshead Two-Factor
      Index)

      _____ Major executives, professionals, proprietors of large concerns
      _____ Lesser executives, professionals, proprietors
      _____ Administrative, small businessmen, minor professionals
      _____ Clerical, technical
      _____ Skilled

_____ Semi-skilled
_____ Unskilled
_____ Housewife
_____ Student
_____ None

h. Head of Household's Education (coded same as f above)

i. Head of Household's Occupation (coded same as g above)

j. Social Class (Hollingshead Two-Factor Index, using education and occupation of head of household) (Five social class categories coded as were raw scores.)

9. WHERE WERE YOU BORN? (both country and region coded)

10. HOW MANY CHILDREN DO YOU HAVE?

_____ None
_____ One or two
_____ Three to Five
_____ Six or more

11. WHEN WERE YOU ADMITTED TO THE HOSPITAL?

_____ Within 1 day
_____ Within 3 days
_____ Within week
_____ (etc.)

12. WHAT WAS THE REASON YOU CAME INTO THE HOS-PITAL? THAT IS, FOR WHAT CONDITION WERE YOU HOS-PITALIZED?

_____

_____

13. IS THIS THE FIRST TIME YOU HAVE BEEN HOSPITALIZED WITH THIS CONDITION? (If not, HOW MANY TIMES?)

_____ Yes, first time
_____ Once before
_____ Two or three times

14. WHAT DOCTOR(S) DID YOU SEE ABOUT IT (PRIOR TO THIS HOSPITALIZATION)? (Record name and determine status, that is, private physician, house staff, research project staff.)

_____ Private physician (coded yes or no)
_____ House staff or clinic (coded yes or no)
_____ Research project staff (coded yes or no)

*15. PEOPLE REACT IN MANY DIFFERENT WAYS TO COMING INTO THE HOSPITAL. HOW DID YOU FEEL ABOUT COMING INTO THE HOSPITAL? (Probe: IS THERE ANYTHING ABOUT COMING INTO THE HOSPITAL THAT WORRIES YOU? IF SO, WHAT?)

Worries mentioned. (All coded yes or no)
_____ Baby's health
_____ Own health
_____ Procedure being done
_____ The experiment
_____ Family worries
_____ Financial worries
_____ General dislike of hospitals
_____ Other worry or general worry

16. WHY DID YOU COME INTO THIS HOSPITAL INSTEAD OF SOME OTHER HOSPITAL?†

17. I'D LIKE TO ASK YOU ABOUT A COUPLE OF OTHER THINGS. I UNDERSTAND THAT YOU ARE TAKING PART IN A RESEARCH STUDY ON INDUCING LABOR.‡
COULD YOU TELL ME A LITTLE ABOUT THE STUDY? (Probe: WHAT IS IT ALL ABOUT? WHAT DO YOU HAVE TO DO IN IT?)

18. WHY DID YOU DECIDE TO PARTICIPATE? (Probes: WHAT REASONS DID YOU GIVE YOURSELF? WHAT FACTORS DID YOU THINK ABOUT?)

Reasons Participated (coded as mentioned or not mentioned)
_____ Wanted or needed the procedure
_____ This was how doctor wanted it done
_____ Self-benefit—medical
_____ Self-benefit—convenience
_____ Self-benefit—other or unspecified
_____ Benefit to science or medicine
_____ Absence of risk, discomfort
_____ Recommended by own doctor
_____ Others felt should participate
_____ Curiosity, interested

* Items 15 thru 23 were asked only during first interviews with labor-induction subjects.
† On this item, as on most open-ended items, space was left on original questionnaire for recording subject's responses.

‡ This item, and the next ones about the research, had to be modified and approached less directly once it was discovered that many subjects were not aware of the research at the time of the first interview (see Chapter Six).

_____ Fear might affect care received
_____ Financial considerations
_____ Other

19. HOW DO YOU FEEL ABOUT THE STUDY? THAT IS—

    a. ARE YOU GLAD YOU ARE IN IT OR NOT? (coded very glad, somewhat glad, a little bit glad, not glad)

    b. ARE YOU INTERESTED IN IT OR EXCITED ABOUT IT? (coded similarly to a)

    c. ARE YOU WORRIED ABOUT IT OR FEARFUL ABOUT IT? (coded similarly to a)

20. HOW DID YOU FIND OUT ABOUT THE STUDY? WHAT DOCTORS DID YOU TALK TO ABOUT IT?

21. WHAT DO YOU THINK OF THE DOCTORS DOING THE STUDY? DO YOU HAVE ANY FEELINGS ABOUT THEM AT THIS TIME?

22. WHY ARE THEY DOING THE STUDY? WHAT DO THEY HOPE TO LEARN?

    _____ Correct response given
    _____ Incorrect response given
    _____ "Don't know"

23. WHY WERE YOU ASKED TO PARTICIPATE, DO YOU HAVE ANY IDEA?

    _____ Know why asked? (coded yes or no)

    If yes, reason given (each coded yes or no)
    _____ To benefit from research
    _____ Because of status (i.e., poor, black, etc.)
    _____ Because needed to be induced
    _____ Because research needed subjects
    _____ Other reason

[This concluded the first interview with labor-induction subjects. Questions 16 through 23 were asked only of those subjects.]

24. WHO (WHAT DOCTOR) SUGGESTED HOSPITALIZATION?

25. WHO ARRANGED FOR THE BED IN THE HOSPITAL? (WHAT DOCTOR?) (Individual private physicians and house staff members coded separately)

26. WAS THERE ANY DOUBT IN YOUR MIND THAT YOU SHOULD GO INTO THE HOSPITAL, OR DID YOU FEEL THAT IT WAS ABSOLUTELY NECESSARY?

27. WHAT ONE THING WORRIED YOU MOST ABOUT GOING INTO THE HOSPITAL? (Probe: DID ANYTHING ELSE WORRY YOU?)

    Any worries reported?
    _____ yes
    _____ no

    If yes, what worried most?
    _____ Finances
    _____ Own condition, pain, etc.
    _____ That baby would be OK
    _____ Things at home, the family
    _____ Research aspects
    _____ Getting proper care
    _____ Other

    All worries reported. (coded mentioned or not mentioned)
    _____ Finances
    _____ Own condition, pain, etc.
    _____ That baby would be OK
    _____ Things at home, the family
    _____ Research aspects
    _____ Getting proper care
    _____ Other

28. AT THE TIME YOU WERE HOSPITALIZED, HOW MUCH WERE YOU WORRIED ABOUT:

    a. THE COSTS INVOLVED IN HOSPITAL—
       _____ A GREAT DEAL?
       _____ A LITTLE BIT?
       _____ NOT AT ALL?

    b. HOW THINGS WOULD GO AT HOME—
       _____ A GREAT DEAL?
       _____ A LITTLE BIT?
       _____ NOT AT ALL?

    c. WHAT WAS TO BE DONE IN THE HOSPITAL—
       _____ A GREAT DEAL?
       _____ A LITTLE BIT?
       _____ NOT AT ALL?

(If worried about what was to be done in hospital, probe: WHAT ASPECT WERE YOU WORRIED ABOUT?

____ Research mentioned

____ Research not mentioned

29. HOW DID YOUR (HUSBAND) (FAMILY) FEEL ABOUT YOUR GOING INTO THE HOSPITAL? WOULD YOU SAY THAT THEY—

____ FELT IT WAS ABSOLUTELY NECESSARY?

____ FELT IT WAS PROBABLY A GOOD IDEA?

____ WERE SOMEWHAT AGAINST THE IDEA?

30. TAKING EVERYTHING INTO CONSIDERATION, WHAT WERE SOME THINGS YOU LIKED *MOST* ABOUT THE CARE AND TREATMENT YOU RECEIVED?

____ liked nothing

____ liked something

What was liked? (each coded as mentioned or not mentioned by subject)

____ Liked everything in general

____ Being induced (labor-induction subjects only)

____ The monitoring, way delivered (labor-induction subjects only)

____ People were nice

____ Other

31. WHAT HAVE YOU LIKED *LEAST?*

____ Disliked nothing

____ Disliked something

What was disliked? (each coded as mentioned or not mentioned by subject)

____ Research

____ Delivery—pain, etc.

____ Blood requests

____ Complaints about the research floor (starvation-abortion subjects only)

____ Food

____ Other

32. WOULD YOU SAY YOUR STAY IN THE HOSPITAL (SO FAR) TURNED OUT BETTER THAN YOU EXPECTED IT TO BE, ABOUT THE SAME, OR WORSE THAN YOU EXPECTED?

____ Better

____ Same

____ Worse

(If better or worse) IN WHAT WAY WAS IT DIFFERENT THAN YOU EXPECTED?

33. CHANGING THE SUBJECT A LITTLE BIT—HOW DOES YOUR (HUSBAND) (FAMILY) FEEL ABOUT THE WAY YOU GENERALLY TAKE CARE OF YOUR HEALTH? (DOES HE) (DO THEY) FEEL THAT YOU ARE GENERALLY:

    ____ TOO CAREFUL ABOUT YOUR HEALTH,
    ____ NOT CAREFUL ENOUGH ABOUT YOUR HEALTH
    ____ ABOUT RIGHT?

34. COMPARED TO MOST PEOPLE, HOW WOULD YOU RATE YOUR CONCERN ABOUT YOUR HEALTH? IN GENERAL, WOULD YOU SAY THAT YOU ARE:

    ____ MORE CONCERNED THAN MOST PEOPLE,
    ____ ABOUT THE SAME AS MOST PEOPLE
    ____ LESS CONCERNED THAN MOST PEOPLE?

35. IN GENERAL, WOULD YOU SAY PEOPLES' CHANCES OF HAVING GOOD HEALTH TODAY ARE BETTER, WORSE, OR ABOUT THE SAME AS THEY WERE 30 YEARS AGO?

    ____ Better
    ____ Worse
    ____ Same

36. (If chances are either better or worse) WHAT ARE SOME OF THE THINGS THAT MAKE CHANCES OF GOOD HEALTH BETTER (OR WORSE) TODAY THAN 30 YEARS AGO? WHO (OR WHAT) IS MAINLY RESPONSIBLE FOR THIS?

    (If better)
    ____ Role of medical research mentioned
    ____ Products of research mentioned
    ____ Other factors only

    (If worse)
    ____ Pollution (coded as mentioned or not mentioned)
    ____ Food, dietary factors (coded as mentioned or not mentioned)
    ____ Other

37. WHY DID YOU COME INTO THIS HOSPITAL INSTEAD OF SOME OTHER HOSPITAL?

    ____ Reason offered
    ____ No reason offered, or alternatives not considered

    Reason mentioned (coded as mentioned or not mentioned)
    ____ Because of doctor
    ____ Because of previous experience
    ____ Because it is research oriented, up-to-date

_____ Because it is a "good hospital," "good care," etc.
_____ Convenience
_____ Other

38. DO YOU THINK THAT HOSPITALS ARE PRETTY MUCH ALIKE WHEN IT COMES TO GIVING PATIENTS THE RIGHT KIND OF CARE, OR NOT?

_____ Yes
_____ No

39. HOW ABOUT THE AMOUNT OF RESEARCH DONE—DO YOU BELIEVE THAT HOSPITALS ARE PRETTY MUCH ALIKE?

_____ Yes
_____ No

40. DO YOU THINK THAT THE AMOUNT OF RESEARCH DONE AT A HOSPITAL HAS ANYTHING TO DO WITH HOW UP-TO-DATE THE HOSPITAL IS?

_____ Yes
_____ No

41. DO YOU THINK THAT HOSPITALS WHERE MUCH RESEARCH IS DONE GENERALLY GIVE THEIR PATIENTS BETTER CARE (THAN OTHER HOSPITALS), ARE THEY ABOUT THE SAME AS OTHER HOSPITALS, OR DO THEY GIVE THEIR PATIENTS WORSE CARE? WHY?

_____ Better
_____ Worse
_____ Same

42. DO YOU BELIEVE THAT THE AMOUNT OF MEDICAL RE-SEARCH DONE HERE IS MORE THAN AT MOST HOSPITALS, LESS THAN AT MOST HOSPITALS, OR ABOUT THE SAME AS AT MOST HOSPITALS?

_____ More here
_____ Less here
_____ Same

43. DO YOU THINK THE EMPHASIS GIVEN RESEARCH AT THIS HOSPITAL IS ABOUT RIGHT, TOO MUCH, OR NOT ENOUGH?

_____ Too much
_____ Not enough
_____ About right

44. DO YOU THINK THE RESEARCH THAT IS DONE HERE HAS ANY EFFECT ON THE QUALITY OF CARE AND TREATMENT PEOPLE RECEIVE? (If so, IN WHAT WAY?)

_____ Yes, has positive effect
_____ Yes, has negative effect
_____ Yes, has mixed effect
_____ No

45. HAS (OR WILL) YOUR HOSPITALIZATION BEEN (BE) MUCH OF A FINANCIAL HARDSHIP? WOULD YOU SAY—

_____ VERY MUCH,
_____ SOMEWHAT OF A HARDSHIP
_____ A SMALL HARDSHIP
_____ NOT A HARDSHIP?

46. HOW HAVE (OR WILL) YOUR HOSPITAL BILLS BEEN (BE) MET— BY YOURSELF AND YOUR FAMILY, BY INSURANCE, BY THE STATE, OR IN SOME OTHER WAY?

_____ By self and family primarily
_____ By self and insurance
_____ Insurance primarily
_____ State (and city) aid
_____ Research funds primarily
_____ Other and other combination

CHANGING THE SUBJECT AGAIN, I UNDERSTAND THAT YOU WERE A SUBJECT IN A STUDY BEING DONE BY DOCTOR _____ ON _____. I WONDER IF WE COULD TALK ABOUT THIS A LITTLE BIT?

47. DID YOU KNOW ABOUT THIS PROJECT (STUDY) BEFORE YOU CAME INTO THE HOSPITAL?

_____ Yes
_____ No (skip to 50)

48. (If yes to 47) DID YOU AGREE TO PARTICIPATE BEFORE AD-MISSION?

_____ Yes
_____ No (skip to 51)

49. (If yes to 48) IF YOU HAD NOT AGREED TO BE A SUBJECT OR PARTICIPATE, WOULD YOU HAVE COME INTO THE HOSPITAL ANYWAY?

_____ Yes
_____ Yes, but only later
_____ No
_____ Do not know
(skip to 51)

50. (If no to 47) DID YOU CONSIDER THE POSSIBILITY THAT YOU MIGHT BE ASKED TO BE A RESEARCH SUBJECT (OR PATIENT) BEFORE YOU CAME INTO THE HOSPITAL?

_____ Yes (If yes, probe: HOW DID YOU FEEL ABOUT IT?)
_____ No

51. LET'S TALK ABOUT HOW YOU BECAME INVOLVED IN THE STUDY. COULD YOU DESCRIBE HOW YOU WERE TOLD ABOUT THE RESEARCH AND HOW THE DOCTOR ASKED YOU TO PARTICIPATE? WHAT DID HE SAY? [This was a key item, and a great deal of probing was used to elicit as complete a description as possible.]

52. WHEN DID YOU FIRST HEAR ABOUT THE STUDY?

_____ Week or more before admission
_____ Two to six days before admission
_____ Day before admission
_____ Day of admission, prior to admission
_____ After admission, before start of research procedures
_____ After the procedure began
_____ Not until procedure had been completed

53. WHO DID YOU TALK TO CONNECTED WITH THE STUDY?

_____ Principal investigator (all response categories coded yes or no)
_____ Other investigator(s)
_____ Nurse
_____ House staff
_____ Private physician
_____ Other

54. HOW MANY DISCUSSIONS DID YOU HAVE WITH THE DOCTORS WORKING ON IT?

_____ None
_____ One
_____ Two
_____ Three or more

55. HOW MUCH TIME (TOTAL) DID THEY SPEND EXPLAINING THE STUDY AND DISCUSSING IT WITH YOU?

____ None
____ Less than 5 minutes
____ 6–15 minutes
____ More than 15 minutes

56. WHEN WERE YOU FIRST ASKED TO PARTICIPATE IN THE STUDY—THE FIRST TIME YOU HEARD ABOUT THE PROJECT, OR LATER?

____ First time
____ Later

57. DID YOU AGREE TO PARTICIPATE THE FIRST TIME YOU WERE ASKED, OR DID YOU WAIT UNTIL LATER TO AGREE?

____ First time
____ Later

58. DID YOU TALK TO ANY DOCTORS NOT CONNECTED WITH THE PROJECT ABOUT THE PROJECT EITHER BEFORE YOU AGREED OR BEFORE YOU TOOK PART IN THE PROJECT?

____ Yes
____ No (skip to 60)

59. (If yes to 58) WHO AND WHEN, AND DID YOU ASK ADVICE?

____ Yes
____ No
(skip to 61)

60. (If no to 58) DID YOU FEEL THE NEED TO TALK TO SUCH A DOCTOR NOT CONNECTED WITH THE RESEARCH? DO YOU THINK THAT WOULD HAVE BEEN HELPFUL TO YOU?

____ Yes
____ No

61. DID YOU DISCUSS WITH OR SEEK ADVICE FROM ANYONE ABOUT WHETHER OR NOT YOU SHOULD PARTICIPATE IN THE STUDY? (If yes, WITH WHOM)

Was advice sought?
____ Yes
____ No
____ Had no opportunity

Source of Advice and Advice Received

a. HUSBAND
    ____ No
    ____ Yes—participation recommended
    ____ Yes—participation not recommended
    ____ Yes—mixed advice offered
    ____ Yes—but no opinion offered

b. OTHER RELATIVES (coded same as a)

c. FRIENDS (coded same as a)

d. OTHER SUBJECTS IN THE STUDY (coded same as a)

e. MEDICAL PEOPLE (OTHER THAN DOCTORS) (coded same as a)

f. ANYONE ELSE (coded same as a)

62. WHEN AND FROM WHOM DID YOU FIND OUT THAT YOU
     WERE (WOULD BE) INVOLVED IN RESEARCH?*

     ____ From doctor before admission
     ____ After admission—from principal investigator
     ____ After admission—from other investigator
     ____ After admission—from other doctor
     ____ After admission—from nurse
     ____ After admission—from me

63. AT WHAT POINT DID YOU SIGN THE CONSENT FORM? (expla-
     nation offered, if necessary)

     ____ Before admission
     ____ After admission, before procedure began
     ____ After procedure began
     ____ Never

64. WHO GAVE YOU THE FORM TO SIGN?

     ____ Principal investigator
     ____ Other investigator
     ____ Nurse

65. WHO EXPLAINED THE MOST ABOUT THE STUDY BEFORE YOU
     ACTUALLY STARTED IN IT?

     ____ Principal investigator
     ____ Other investigator

* Items 62–66 were added to the questionnaire after the discovery of *unaware* labor-induction
subjects showed these matters to be important.

_____ Nurse
_____ House staff
_____ Private physician
_____ Consent form
_____ Other
_____ No one

66. OVERALL—BOTH BEFORE AND DURING THE STUDY—WHO EXPLAINED OR TOLD YOU THE MOST ABOUT THE STUDY? (coded the same as 65 with the interviewer added as a response category)

67. HOW DIFFICULT WOULD YOU SAY THE DECISION WAS ON WHETHER OR NOT TO PARTICIPATE?

_____ NOT AT ALL DIFFICULT (Skip to 69)
_____ SOMEWHAT DIFFICULT
_____ VERY DIFFICULT

68. (If had some difficulty) WHAT MADE THE DECISION DIFFICULT?

69. WHEN YOU WERE ASKED TO PARTICIPATE—DID IT OCCUR TO YOU TO SAY NO?

_____ Yes
_____ No

70. DID YOU GIVE SERIOUS CONSIDERATION TO REFUSING?

_____ Yes
_____ No

71. HOW MUCH THOUGHT DID YOU GIVE TO THE DECISION—DID YOU MAKE UP YOUR MIND IMMEDIATELY, OR DID YOU GIVE IT *SOME* THOUGHT, OR A *GREAT DEAL* OF THOUGHT?

_____ Agreed immediately
_____ Gave it some thought
_____ Gave it a great deal of thought

72. DID YOU FEEL THAT YOU HAD ALL THE INFORMATION YOU NEEDED OR WANTED IN ORDER TO MAKE YOUR DECISION?

_____ Yes
_____ No (Probe: WHAT OTHER INFORMATION COULD YOU HAVE USED?)

73. WERE THERE ANY ASPECTS OF THE STUDY THAT YOU FELT
     THAT YOU DID NOT UNDERSTAND?

     ____ Yes (If so, WHAT WERE THEY?)
     ____ No

74. BEFORE THE RESEARCH STARTED, HOW WELL DID YOU FEEL
     YOU UNDERSTOOD: (all response categories same as a)

     a. WHAT WAS TO BE DONE?
         ____ UNDERSTOOD COMPLETELY
         ____ UNDERSTOOD FAIRLY WELL
         ____ DIDN'T UNDERSTAND VERY WELL
         ____ DIDN'T UNDERSTAND AT ALL

     b. ANY RISKS THAT MIGHT BE INVOLVED?

     c. THE POTENTIAL BENEFITS TO YOURSELF?

     d. THE POTENTIAL BENEFITS TO SCIENCE—WHAT THEY
         HOPED TO LEARN?

     e. YOUR ROLE—WHAT WAS EXPECTED OF YOU?

     f. THE TECHNICAL ASPECTS OF THE RESEARCH?

75. HOW DID YOU FEEL ABOUT BEING ASKED TO PARTICIPATE?

     ____ Pleased or glad
     ____ Worried or fearful
     ____ Indifferent
     ____ Mixed feelings

SO FAR WE HAVE BEEN TALKING ABOUT YOUR DECISION TO PAR-
TICIPATE IN THE STUDY—NOW LET'S TALK ABOUT THE STUDY IT-
SELF.

76. WHAT WAS (IS) THE PROJECT ABOUT? (Probes: WHAT DID (DO)
     YOU HAVE TO DO? WHAT WAS (WILL BE) DONE THAT IN-
     VOLVED(S) YOU?)

77. BEFORE THE STUDY BEGAN, DID YOU KNOW (OR WAS IT
     YOUR UNDERSTANDING):*

     a. THAT A NEW DRUG WAS TO BE USED OR MIGHT BE USED
         OR NOT? (this and following items coded yes or no)

* Items 77 and 78 were added after several interviews were done because of weaknesses in the
original questionnaire, particularly the difficulty in confidently assessing subjects' knowledge
of the labor-induction study solely on the basis of item 76.

    b. THAT THEY WERE USING MORE THAN ONE DRUG OR NOT?

    c. HOW THE DRUG WAS TO BE GIVEN?

    d. WHAT KIND OF DRUG IT WAS (OR ANYTHING ABOUT IT)

    e. WHAT DRUG THEY WOULD ACTUALLY USE? (Probe to determine if blind aspect understood.)

    f. IF ANY RISKS WERE INVOLVED OR NOT?

    g. IF THEY WERE GOING TO DO ANY SPECIAL MONITORING OR OBSERVING OF YOUR LABOR OR NOT?

    h. IF THEY WERE GOING TO DO ANY SPECIAL OBSERVING OR STUDYING OF THE BABY AFTER IT WAS BORN?

    i. IF THEY WERE GOING TO DO ANY SPECIAL OR EXTRA TESTS (LIKE BLOOD TESTS) ON YOU OR NOT?

    j. HOW LONG THEY WOULD CONTINUE TO TRY IT IF IT DIDN'T WORK AT FIRST?

    k. WHAT WOULD HAPPEN IF IT (THE DRUG) DIDN'T WORK?

78. IF YOU HAD DECIDED THAT YOU DID NOT WANT TO BE IN THE STUDY, WHAT WOULD THEY HAVE DONE?

    _____ Induced the regular way
    _____ Waited for labor
    _____ Waited for induction
    _____ Don't know

79. WHY DO YOU THINK THAT *YOU* WERE ASKED TO BE A SUBJECT IN THIS RESEARCH?

    _____ Because of specific benefits received
    _____ Because of general benefits
    _____ Because needed to be induced
    _____ Status reason (i.e., poor or black)
    _____ Met research criteria or to help the researchers
    _____ Don't know

80. WHY DID YOU AGREE TO PARTICIPATE? (Probes: WHAT REASONS DID YOU GIVE YOURSELF? WHAT FACTORS DID YOU CONSIDER? ANY OTHER REASONS?)

Factors mentioned (all coded as mentioned or not mentioned)

    a. This was how doctor wanted it done

    b. Self-benefit—medical

    c. Self-benefit—convenience

    d. Self-benefit—other or unspecified

    e. Benefit to science

    f. Absence of risks

    g. Recommended by own doctor

    h. Others felt should do so

    i. Curiosity, interest

    j. To get better care, because it would affect care

    k. Financial considerations

    l. Other

Other factors considered (all coded as mentioned or not mentioned)

    a. Risks

    b. Discomfort

    c. Other

81. a. AT THE TIME YOU DECIDED TO PARTICIPATE—DID YOU THINK THAT THE RESEARCH WOULD BE OF ANY MEDICAL BENEFIT TO YOURSELF?

    _____ Yes (Probe: IN WHAT WAY?)
    _____ Maybe (Probe: IN WHAT WAY?)
    _____ No

  b. IN DECIDING TO PARTICIPATE, HOW MUCH THOUGHT DID YOU GIVE TO THE FACTOR OF PERSONAL BENEFIT?

    _____ NONE
    _____ VERY LITTLE
    _____ SOME
    _____ A GREAT DEAL

  c. HOW IMPORTANT A FACTOR WAS IT IN YOUR DECISION?

    _____ NOT A FACTOR
    _____ NOT VERY IMPORTANT
    _____ SOMEWHAT IMPORTANT
    _____ VERY IMPORTANT

  d. (If saw medical benefit present) WHAT TREATMENT WOULD THEY HAVE USED IF YOU HAD DECIDED NOT TO PAR-

TICIPATE IN THE RESEARCH? WHAT TREATMENT OPTIONS
DID YOU HAVE?

_____ Option was to wait for labor
_____ Option was to be induced another way
_____ Did not think had an option
_____ Did not know about options

82. a. WERE THERE ANY RISKS OF COMPLICATIONS INVOLVED?

_____ Yes (Probe: WHAT RISKS?)
_____ No

b. IN DECIDING TO PARTICIPATE, HOW MUCH THOUGHT DID
YOU GIVE TO RISKS? (same response categories as 81b)

c. HOW IMPORTANT WERE RISKS AS A FACTOR IN YOUR DE-
CISION? (same response categories as 81c)

83. a. DID YOU BELIEVE THAT THERE WOULD BE ANY PAIN OR
DISCOMFORT INVOLVED IN THE STUDY?

_____ Yes
_____ Maybe
_____ No

_____ (If expected discomfort) WHAT SORT OF PAIN AND DIS-
COMFORT DID YOU EXPECT?

_____ A GREAT DEAL OF PAIN OR DISCOMFORT
_____ SOME
_____ VERY MINOR OR TEMPORARY PAIN OR DIS-
COMFORT

b. HOW MUCH THOUGHT DID YOU GIVE TO PAIN OR DIS-
COMFORT IN DECIDING TO PARTICIPATE? (same response
categories as 81b)

c. HOW IMPORTANT WAS PAIN AND DISCOMFORT AS A
FACTOR IN YOUR DECISION? (same response categories as 81c)

84. a. DID YOU BELIEVE THAT THE STUDY WOULD MEAN ANY
INCONVENIENCE TO YOU?

_____ Yes
_____ No

_____ (If yes) WHAT SORT OF INCONVENIENCE?

_____ SMALL OR MINOR INCONVENIENCE
_____ A GREAT DEAL OR MAJOR INCONVENIENCE

b. HOW MUCH THOUGHT DID YOU GIVE TO INCONVENIENCE IN DECIDING TO PARTICIPATE? (same categories as 81b)

c. HOW IMPORTANT WAS INCONVENIENCE AS A FACTOR IN YOUR DECISION? (same categories as 81c)

85. a. DID YOU BELIEVE THAT THE RESEARCH MIGHT PRODUCE KNOWLEDGE THAT MIGHT HELP YOU OR YOUR LOVED ONES SOMETIME IN THE FUTURE?

____ Yes
____ No

b. HOW MUCH THOUGHT DID YOU GIVE TO THIS? (same categories as 81b)

c. HOW IMPORTANT IN YOUR DECISION WOULD YOU SAY THIS FACTOR WAS? (same categories as 81c)

86. a. WERE YOU AT ALL AFRAID BECAUSE YOU DID NOT KNOW WHAT TO EXPECT?

____ Yes
____ No
____ (If Yes) TO WHAT EXTENT? WERE YOU
____ A LITTLE BIT AFRAID,
____ SOMEWHAT AFRAID
____ VERY MUCH AFRAID

b. HOW MUCH THOUGHT DID YOU GIVE TO THIS (FEAR), IN DECIDING TO PARTICIPATE? (same categories as 81b)

c. HOW IMPORTANT WAS THIS AS A FACTOR IN YOUR DECISION TO PARTICIPATE? (same categories as 81c)

87. a. DID YOU BELIEVE THAT BEING IN THIS RESEARCH (OR REFUSING TO PARTICIPATE) MIGHT AFFECT THE CARE YOU WOULD RECEIVE OR THE WAY YOU WERE TREATED WHILE IN THE HOSPITAL?

____ Yes (Probe: IN WHAT WAY?)
____ No

b. HOW MUCH THOUGHT DID YOU GIVE TO THIS IN DECIDING TO PARTICIPATE? (same categories as 81b)

c. HOW IMPORTANT WAS THIS AS A FACTOR IN YOUR DECISION? (same categories as 81c)

88. a. DID YOU BELIEVE THAT IT WOULD BE AN INTERESTING EXPERIENCE? THAT IS, WERE YOU CURIOUS WHAT IT WOULD BE LIKE?

_____ Yes
_____ No

_____ (If Yes) WERE YOU:

_____ A LITTLE BIT CURIOUS OR INTERESTED,
_____ SOMEWHAT CURIOUS OR INTERESTED
_____ VERY CURIOUS OR INTERESTED

 b. HOW MUCH THOUGHT DID YOU GIVE TO THIS IN DECIDING TO PARTICIPATE? (same categories as 81b)

 c. HOW IMPORTANT WAS THIS AS A FACTOR IN YOUR DECISION TO PARTICIPATE? (same categories as 81c)

89. a. DID THE DOCTOR(S) DOING THE RESEARCH FEEL STRONGLY THAT YOU SHOULD PARTICIPATE?

_____ Yes
_____ No

_____ (If yes) TO WHAT EXTENT? WOULD YOU SAY THEY FELT FAIRLY STRONGLY OR VERY STRONGLY THAT YOU SHOULD?

_____ Fairly strongly
_____ Very strongly

 b. HOW MUCH DID YOU THINK ABOUT THIS IN DECIDING TO PARTICIPATE? (same categories as 81b)

 c. HOW IMPORTANT WAS THIS AS A FACTOR IN YOUR DECISION TO PARTICIPATE? (same categories as 81c)

90. a. DID YOU BELIEVE THAT THERE WOULD BE ANY FINANCIAL BENEFIT OR SPECIAL ACCOMMODATIONS IF YOU PARTICIPATED?

_____ Yes
_____ Maybe
_____ No

_____ (If yes or maybe) OF WHAT SORT—FINANCIAL BENEFITS, SPECIAL ACCOMMODATIONS, OR BOTH?

_____ Financial benefits
_____ Special accomodations
_____ Both

b.   HOW MUCH DID YOU THINK ABOUT THIS IN DECIDING TO
     PARTICIPATE? (same categories as 81b)

c.   HOW IMPORTANT WAS THIS AS A FACTOR IN YOUR DE-
     CISION? (same categories as 81c)

91. a.   DID YOU BELIEVE THAT IT WOULD HELP THE RE-
          SEARCHER(S) IF YOU PARTICIPATED?

          _____ Yes
          _____ No

          _____ (If Yes) IN WHAT WAY WOULD IT HELP THEM?

          _____ Career
          _____ Help science
          _____ Both
          _____ Other, help them help others

     b.   HOW MUCH DID YOU THINK ABOUT THIS IN DECIDING TO
          PARTICIPATE? (same categories as 81b)

     c.   HOW IMPORTANT WAS THIS AS A FACTOR IN YOUR DE-
          CISION? (same categories as 81c)

92. a.   DID YOU BELIEVE THAT YOUR PARTICIPATION MIGHT
          HELP TO ADVANCE MEDICAL SCIENCE?

          _____ Definitely
          _____ Possibly
          _____ No

     b.   HOW MUCH DID YOU THINK ABOUT THIS IN DECIDING TO
          PARTICIPATE? (same categories as 81b)

     c.   HOW IMPORTANT WAS THIS AS A FACTOR IN YOUR DE-
          CISION? (same categories as 81c)

93. a.   WHAT DID YOU KNOW OR HOW MUCH DID YOU KNOW
          ABOUT THE DOCTOR(S) DOING THE RESEARCH BEFORE
          THE RESEARCH STARTED? [After giving a free response, subjects
          were asked:] WOULD YOU SAY YOU KNEW A GREAT DEAL
          ABOUT THEM, SOME, A LITTLE, OR NOTHING ABOUT
          THEM?

          _____ A great deal
          _____ Some
          _____ A little
          _____ Nothing

    b. HOW MUCH DID YOU THINK ABOUT THIS IN DECIDING TO PARTICIPATE? (same categories as 81b)

    c. HOW IMPORTANT WAS THIS AS A FACTOR IN YOUR DECISION? (same categories as 81c)

94. LOOKING BACK ON IT NOW, WHAT FACTORS WOULD YOU SAY WERE THE MOST IMPORTANT IN YOUR DECIDING TO PARTICIPATE? (Probe: ANY OTHER FACTORS YOU CONSIDERED?) (all responses coded same as a)

    a. This was how doctor wanted it done.

        ____ Major reason (designated by subject)
        ____ Other reason mentioned
        ____ Not mentioned

    b. Self-benefit—medical

    c. Self-benefit—convenience

    d. Self-benefit—other or unspecified

    e. Benefit to science (or to others)

    f. Absence of risks

    g. Recommended by own doctor

    h. Others felt should do so

    i. Curiosity, interest

    j. To get better care; because it would affect care

    k. Financial considerations

    l. Knowledge of the researcher(s)

95. DO YOU THINK YOU WOULD HAVE FELT BAD (OR GUILTY) ABOUT IT IF YOU HAD DECIDED NOT TO PARTICIPATE AS A SUBJECT?

    ____ Yes (Probe: WHY?)
    ____ No

96. WHAT DO YOU THINK OF THE DOCTOR(S) DOING THE RESEARCH? COULD YOU DESCRIBE YOUR FEELINGS ABOUT THEM?

    ____ Positive
    ____ Negative
    ____ Mixed, neither

97. HOW DID IT GO? WAS THE EXPERIENCE PRETTY MUCH AS YOU EXPECTED IT TO BE OR WAS IT DIFFERENT? [Items 97–103 were for respondents who had already acted as subjects in a project. It turned out that all respondents interviewed fell into this category.]

    ____ Same as expected (skip to 98b)
    ____ Different

(If Different, Probe: HOW MUCH DIFFERENT WAS IT—

    ____ A LITTLE BIT DIFFERENT
    ____ SOMEWHAT DIFFERENT
    ____ VERY MUCH DIFFERENT

98. a. (If different) IN WHAT WAYS WAS IT DIFFERENT THAN YOU EXPECTED IT TO BE?

    b. WAS IT MORE OR LESS INTERESTING THAN YOU EXPECTED, OR THE SAME?

        ____ More interesting
        ____ Same
        ____ Less interesting

    c. WAS THERE MORE OR LESS DISCOMFORT THAN YOU EXPECTED, OR THE SAME? (coded same as b)

    d. WAS THERE MORE OR LESS INCONVENIENCE THAN YOU EXPECTED, OR THE SAME? (coded same as b)

    e. WAS YOUR RELATIONSHIP WITH THE RESEARCHER(S) LIKE YOU EXPECTED OR WAS IT DIFFERENT?

        ____ Like expected
        ____ Different

        ____ (If different) HOW WAS IT DIFFERENT?

        ____ Better
        ____ Worse
        ____ Unspecified

99. WERE YOU SATISFIED WITH THE ROLE YOU PLAYED OR WOULD YOU HAVE PREFERRED A MORE OR LESS ACTIVE ROLE? (Role: what they wanted you to do)

    ____ Prefer more active role
    ____ Satisfied
    ____ Prefer less active role

100. DO YOU FEEL THAT YOU RECEIVED ANY BENEFIT FROM THIS PROJECT? (If yes, probe: IN WHAT WAY?)

    _____ Yes, medical benefit
    _____ Yes, learned or had interesting experience
    _____ Yes, other
    _____ No

101. DO YOU FEEL THAT YOU RECEIVED ANY HARM FROM THE PROJECT?

    _____ Yes
    _____ Possibly
    _____ No

102. DID YOU THINK ABOUT STOPPING YOUR INVOLVEMENT IN THE STUDY AT ANY TIME?

    _____ Yes
    _____ No (skip to 104)

103. a. (If yes to 102) HOW SERIOUSLY DID YOU THINK ABOUT IT, OR DID YOU ACTUALLY DO IT? (If didn't actually do it) WOULD YOU SAY THAT YOU GAVE IT *SOME* THOUGHT OR THAT YOU GAVE IT *SERIOUS* THOUGHT?

    _____ Gave it some thought
    _____ Gave it serious thought
    _____ Actually did it

    b. (If thought about it or did it) WHY DID YOU (DO IT) (THINK ABOUT IT)?

    c. (If thought about it or did it) DID YOU TALK TO ANYONE ABOUT IT? WHO? WHAT DID THEY SAY?

104. a. HAVE YOU BEEN ASKED TO BE A SUBJECT IN ANY OTHER PROJECTS DURING YOUR STAY IN THE HOSPITAL?

    _____ Yes
    _____ No (skip to 105)

    b. (If yes) HOW MANY?

    c. (If yes to 104a) DID YOU AGREE TO BE A SUBJECT IN ALL PROJECTS?

    _____ Yes—all
    _____ Yes—some
    _____ No

d. (If yes to 104a) WERE THE SAME RESEARCHERS INVOLVED AS IN THE PROJECT WE HAVE BEEN DISCUSSING?

105. HAVE YOU HAD ANY OTHER EXPERIENCES WITH RESEARCH DURING YOUR STAY IN THE HOSPITAL?

____ Yes
____ Maybe
____ No

106. HAVE YOU EVER BEEN A SUBJECT IN ANY OTHER PROJECTS BEFORE THIS HOSPITALIZATION?

____ Yes (Probe: WHAT WAS IT?)
____ No

107. IN GENERAL, DO YOU THINK THAT PEOPLE HAVE AN OBLIGATION TO COOPERATE WHENEVER A DOCTOR ASKS THEM TO ACT AS RESEARCH SUBJECTS?

____ Yes
____ Yes, conditionally
____ No

108. ON THE BASIS OF YOUR EXPERIENCE (THUS FAR), WHAT FACTORS WOULD YOU SAY ONE SHOULD CONSIDER BEFORE DECIDING TO BE A RESEARCH SUBJECT? (Probe: IF ONE OF YOUR FRIENDS WERE ASKED TO BE IN A RESEARCH PROJECT, WHAT SORTS OF THINGS WOULD YOU ADVISE HER TO FIND OUT ABOUT?)

Factors which should be considered. (all coded as mentioned or not mentioned)

a. Self–benefits

b. Risks

c. Pain, discomfort

d. Inconvenience

e. Benefit to science

f. Treatment in hospital

g. General—"Find out everything"

h. Other

109. IF YOU WERE ASKED TO PARTICIPATE IN A PROJECT SIMILAR TO THIS ONE IN THE FUTURE, HOW WILLING WOULD YOU BE? WOULD YOU BE—

    ____ VERY WILLING,
    ____ SOMEWHAT WILLING,
    ____ SOMEWHAT UNWILLING
    ____ VERY UNWILLING

110. HAS YOUR EXPERIENCE (THUS FAR) IN THIS RESEARCH PROJECT CHANGED, IN ANY WAY, THE WAY YOU FEEL ABOUT DOCTORS?

    ____ Positive change
    ____ Negative change
    ____ Mixed change
    ____ No change

111. HAS IT CHANGED YOUR FEELINGS ABOUT THIS HOSPITAL? (same response categories as 110)

112. HAS IT CHANGED YOUR FEELINGS ABOUT MEDICAL RESEARCH? (same response categories as 110)

113. IN GENERAL, DO YOU THINK THAT BEING A SUBJECT IN RESEARCH HAS ANY EFFECT ON A PERSON'S CHANCES OF GETTING WELL?

    ____ Yes—positive effect
    ____ Yes—negative effect
    ____ Yes—qualified
    ____ No

114. IN GENERAL, WHO DO YOU THINK BENEFITS FROM MOST MEDICAL RESEARCH—SUBJECTS OR FUTURE PATIENTS?

    ____ Subjects
    ____ Future patients
    ____ Situational (e.g., "It depends upon the research.")
    ____ Both

115. HOW ABOUT RESEARCHERS—DO THEY BENEFIT?

    ____ Yes, career
    ____ Yes, helps scientific knowledge
    ____ Yes, other
    ____ Yes, unspecified
    ____ No

116. CHANGING THE SUBJECT A BIT—GENERALLY, WHEN YOU
     ARE ILL AND SEE A DOCTOR, DO YOU DEMAND TO KNOW ALL
     THE DETAILS OF WHAT IS BEING DONE TO YOU?

     _____ Yes
     _____ No

117. GENERALLY, WHEN YOU ARE GETTING TREATMENT FROM A
     DOCTOR, HOW WELL DO YOU USUALLY UNDERSTAND WHAT
     THEY ARE DOING AND WHY THEY ARE DOING IT? DO YOU—

     _____ USUALLY UNDERSTAND COMPLETELY
     _____ USUALLY UNDERSTAND FAIRLY WELL
     _____ HAVE SOME UNDERSTANDING, BUT MUCH IS NOT
           CLEAR
     _____ HAVE VERY LITTLE UNDERSTANDING
     _____ USUALLY UNDERSTAND NOTHING OF WHAT THE
           DOCTOR IS DOING

118. DO YOU THINK YOU UNDERSTAND (UNDERSTOOD) WHAT
     THE DOCTOR(S) (WILL DO) (DID) IN CONNECTION WITH THE
     RESEARCH THIS TIME BETTER THAN YOU USUALLY UNDER-
     STAND WHAT DOCTORS ARE DOING, NOT AS WELL AS USUAL,
     OR ABOUT THE SAME? WOULD YOU SAY THAT YOU—

     _____ UNDERSTOOD MUCH BETTER THAN USUAL
     _____ UNDERSTOOD SOMEWHAT BETTER THAN USUAL
     _____ SAME AS USUAL
     _____ SOMEWHAT LESS WELL THAN USUAL
     _____ MUCH LESS WELL THAN USUAL

119. CHANGING THE SUBJECT A BIT AGAIN—DO YOU THINK THAT
     YOU HAVE MORE FAITH IN MEDICINE THAN MOST PEOPLE,
     LESS THAN MOST PEOPLE, OR ABOUT THE SAME?

     _____ More
     _____ Same
     _____ Less

120. DO YOU THINK YOU TRUST DOCTORS MORE THAN MOST
     PEOPLE, LESS THAN MOST PEOPLE, OR ABOUT THE SAME AS
     MOST PEOPLE?

     _____ More
     _____ Same
     _____ Less

121. DO YOU BELIEVE THAT MOST DOCTORS ARE MORE INTERESTED IN THE WELFARE OF THEIR PATIENTS THAN ANYTHING ELSE?

    _____ Yes
    _____ No (Probe: WHY? WHAT ARE THEY INTERESTED IN?)

122. DO YOU THINK THAT A DOCTOR'S DOING RESEARCH HAS ANY EFFECT ON HIS INTEREST IN HIS PATIENTS?

    _____ Yes (Probe: IN WHAT WAY?)
    _____ Maybe (Probe: IN WHAT WAY?)
    _____ No
    _____ Don't know

123. DO YOU BELIEVE IN TRYING OUT DIFFERENT DOCTORS TO FIND ONE YOU THINK WILL GIVE YOU THE BEST CARE?

    _____ Yes
    _____ No

124. DO YOU FIND IT HARD TO GIVE IN AND GO TO BED WHEN YOU ARE SICK?

    _____ Yes
    _____ No

125. DO YOU TRY TO GET UP TOO SOON AFTER YOU HAVE BEEN SICK?

    _____ Yes
    _____ No

126. WHEN YOU ARE SICK AND NEED TO SEE A DOCTOR, WHERE DO YOU GENERALLY GO TO GET CARE?

    _____ Private physician (WHO?)
    _____ Medical school faculty member
    _____ Hospital clinic
    _____ Hospital emergency room
    _____ Other

127. DO YOU HAVE DOUBTS ABOUT SOME THINGS DOCTORS SAY THEY CAN DO FOR YOU IN GENERAL?

    _____ OFTEN
    _____ OCCASIONALLY
    _____ No

128.   DO YOU BELIEVE THAT MOST DOCTORS CHARGE TOO MUCH?

_____ Yes
_____ Sometimes
_____ No

FINALLY, TO FINISH UP THE INTERVIEW, I HAVE A FEW QUES-
TIONS ABOUT YOUR EVERYDAY LIFE AND YOUR BACKGROUND.

129.   DOES EVERYONE IN YOUR FAMILY USUALLY DO WHAT (YOU)
       (THE HEAD OF THE HOUSEHOLD) SAY(S) WITHOUT QUES-
       TIONS?

_____ Yes
_____ No

130.   DOES YOUR FAMILY USUALLY EAT THE EVENING MEAL
       TOGETHER?

_____ Yes
_____ No

131.   IN YOUR FAMILY, DO YOU THINK THE OLD-TIME TRADITIONS
       AND CUSTOMS ARE IMPORTANT?

_____ Yes
_____ No

132.   ABOUT HOW MANY PEOPLE ARE THERE WHOM YOU
       CONSIDER TO BE CLOSE FRIENDS (A PERSON TO WHOM YOU
       CAN TELL WHAT IS ON YOUR MIND)? (coded 0 through 11 or more)

133.   GENERALLY, ABOUT HOW OFTEN DO YOU GET TOGETHER
       WITH FRIENDS AND RELATIVES? THINGS LIKE GOING OUT
       TOGETHER OR VISITING IN EACH OTHER'S HOMES?

_____ MORE THAN ONCE A WEEK
_____ ABOUT ONCE A WEEK
_____ A FEW TIMES A MONTH
_____ ONCE A MONTH
_____ LESS THAN ONCE A MONTH

134.   HAVE YOU EVER VOLUNTEERED TO GIVE BLOOD?

_____ Yes
_____ No

(If yes) HOW OFTEN?

____ RARELY
____ OCCASIONALLY
____ REGULARLY

135. HAVE YOU EVER VOLUNTEERED FOR ANY KIND OF RESEARCH
      OTHER THAN MEDICAL?

      ____ Yes (Probe: COULD YOU DESCRIBE IT?)
      ____ No

136. WHERE WAS YOUR FATHER BORN? IN WHAT COUNTRY?

      ____ U.S.
      ____ Other American
      ____ European
      ____ Other

137. WHERE WAS YOUR MOTHER BORN? IN WHAT COUNTRY? (same
      response categories as 136)

138. WHAT WAS THE HIGHEST GRADE IN SCHOOL COMPLETED BY
      YOUR FATHER? (same response categories as 8f)

139. (When subject was 18–20 years old) WHAT WAS HIS USUAL OCCU-
      PATION? (same occupational categories as 8g)

140. IN WHAT RELIGION WERE YOU RAISED AND WHAT IS YOUR
      PRESENT RELIGION?

      a. Religion in which raised

          ____ Protestant
          ____ Roman Catholic
          ____ Jewish
          ____ Other
          ____ No religious preference

      b. Present preference
          ____ (Same categories as 140a)

141. DO YOU CONSIDER YOURSELF:

      ____ DEEPLY RELIGIOUS
      ____ MODERATELY RELIGIOUS
      ____ LARGELY INDIFFERENT TO RELIGION
      ____ BASICALLY OPPOSED TO RELIGION

142. ARE YOU AFFILIATED WITH ANY CHURCH OR RELIGIOUS GROUP?

_____ Yes
_____ No

143. ABOUT HOW OFTEN DO YOU ATTEND RELIGIOUS SERVICES—

_____ ONCE A WEEK OR MORE OFTEN
_____ TWO OR THREE TIMES A MONTH
_____ ONCE A MONTH
_____ A FEW TIMES A YEAR OR LESS
_____ NEVER

144. DO YOU BELONG TO ANY ORGANIZATIONS OR GROUPS WITHIN THE CHURCH?

_____ Yes, more than one
_____ Yes, one
_____ No (skip to 146)

145. (If yes to 144) HOW OFTEN DO YOU USUALLY ATTEND MEETINGS—

_____ REGULARLY
_____ SOMETIMES
_____ RARELY
_____ NEVER

146. DO YOU NOW BELONG TO ANY CLUBS, LODGES, UNIONS, OR ORGANIZED GROUPS?

_____ Yes
_____ No (skip to 148)

(If yes) HOW MANY?

_____ One
_____ Two or three
_____ Four or more

147. (If yes to 146) HOW OFTEN DO YOU USUALLY ATTEND MEETINGS—

_____ REGULARLY
_____ SOMETIMES
_____ RARELY
_____ NEVER

148. IN YOUR GROUP OR CHURCH ACTIVITIES, WHEN THINGS NEED TO BE DONE ARE YOU MORE LIKELY THAN MOST PEOPLE TO VOLUNTEER YOUR SERVICES, LESS LIKELY THAN MOST PEOPLE, OR ABOUT THE SAME AS MOST PEOPLE?

_____ More likely
_____ Same
_____ Less likely

149. DO YOU CONSIDER YOURSELF TO BE THE CHIEF BREADWINNER (SOURCE OF INCOME) FOR THE FAMILY?

_____ Yes
_____ No

(If no) WHICH MEMBER OF THE HOUSEHOLD IS THE CHIEF BREADWINNER?

_____ No one
_____ Spouse
_____ Parent
_____ Other relative
_____ Other

150. COULD YOU TELL ME HOW MUCH THE CHIEF BREADWINNER (YOU) EARN(S)? (specify amount and period) (coded in thousand dollar increments)

151. COULD YOU GIVE ME YOUR BEST ESTIMATE OF ALL THE INCOME EARNED OR RECEIVED BY MEMBERS OF YOUR HOUSEHOLD DURING THE PAST YEAR? (coded in thousand dollar increments)

152. WHICH OF THE FOLLOWING WAS THE SINGLE MOST IMPORTANT SOURCE OF INCOME FOR THE HOUSEHOLD DURING THE PAST YEAR—

_____ WAGES, SALARY, COMMISSIONS
_____ OWN BUSINESS OR PROFESSIONAL PRACTICE
_____ INTEREST OR DIVIDENDS ON SAVINGS, STOCKS, OR BONDS, OR RENTAL INCOME
_____ UNEMPLOYMENT COMPENSATION
_____ PUBLIC ASSISTANCE OR WELFARE PAYMENTS
_____ OTHER

153. HOW MANY PERSONS ARE DEPENDENT UPON THIS INCOME FOR AT LEAST HALF THEIR SUPPORT? (both the number and an income per person coded)

INDEX